Historical Diseases from a Modern Perspective

James A. Shaw

Historical Diseases from a Modern Perspective

The American Experience

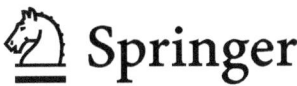 Springer

James A. Shaw
Clinical Professor (Retired)
SUNY Upstate Medical University
Syracuse, NY, USA

ISBN 978-3-031-52345-8   ISBN 978-3-031-52346-5   (eBook)
https://doi.org/10.1007/978-3-031-52346-5

This Springer imprint is published by the registered company Springer Nature Switzerland AG
The registered company address is: Gewerbestrasse 11, 6330 Cham, Switzerland

If disposing of this product, please recycle the paper.

For my wife, Nancy, whose companionship and love have brought joy to my life.

"Fortunate is he whose mind has the power to probe the causes of things and trample underfoot all terrors and inexorable fate."

Virgil

Introduction

Note to Readers

James A. Shaw

Despite being a medical doctor, student of history, and fan of historical novels, I am often stumped when an author refers to *Ague*, *Ship Fever*, *Blue Death*, *Quincy*, *Scarlatina*, *French Pox*, *Consumption*, *Congestive Fever*, *Black Plague*, *Bronze John*, *Breakbone Fever*, etc., and am forced to make a trip to the Internet for clarification.[1] Not infrequently, ancient diseases and/or symptoms are inadequately or incorrectly described in historical novels and are often afforded superficial context in history books, where they are referred to somewhat peripherally. It is my hope that this short book will provide an informative reference for readers who are similarly puzzled when confronted with an unfamiliar disease in a novel or book of history.

Like COVID-19, the impact that yellow fever, malaria, smallpox, measles, polio, cholera, and 1918 pandemic influenza, among many others, had on Americans was profound and, in some cases, overwhelming. U.S. military campaigns, starting with smallpox in the Revolutionary War, dysentery in the Civil War, influenza in WWI, malaria in WWII, opioids in Vietnam, and sexually transmitted diseases across all wars, markedly impacted troop strength and preparedness. In many instances American physician-scientists identified the origins, transmission vectors, and cures for these diseases, which is fascinating history in and of itself.

I suspect that most readers are vaguely aware of the devastating impact of bubonic plague over the ages in the Old World. But how many realize a plague epidemic occurred in San Francisco in 1900, fortuitously controlled before becoming a pandemic by epidemiologists who identified rats as the reservoir of disease and

---

[1] For example, David Grann refers to "saffron scourge," "bloody flux," "breakbone fever," "blue death," and "ship's fever" within the first chapter of his book, *The Wager: A Tale of Shipwreck, Mutiny and Murder* (Doubleday, New York, NY; 2023).

fleas as the communicating vector? (A thriller story in its own right!) How many are aware that a few cases of plague still occur in the United States every year and that squirrels are a persistent reservoir of the disease?

How many are aware that smallpox nearly annihilated the Native American population and decimated Revolutionary War soldiers, polio was every parent's nightmare, cholera epidemics plagued U.S. cities, chicken pox "parties" were once common, and the 1918 influenza pandemic may have started in the United States and may have shortened the duration of WWI? I suspect very few realize that leprosy occurred in the United States or are aware of the horrors of pre-antibiotic treatment of this debilitating disease. How many know that the Centers of Disease Control and Prevention (CDC) had its inception in 1946, with one of its foundational missions to stop the spread of malaria across the nation?

****

The history of diseases is intrinsically fascinating and may be of particular interest to readers in light of the recent COVID-19 pandemic. Most diseases have many interconnected aspects of historical importance—medical, social, economic, and political—which I have tried to condense into a few summary paragraphs for each disease covered. Intrinsic to such brevity is the risk of oversimplification, which I recognize as a potential concern. That said, any subject the reader finds of interest can be further clarified by an Internet search using any of the references listed at the end of each section, among many others.

The cited references were principally selected for their ready Internet availability, authoritative authorship, and content written at a level understandable by a lay audience. They represent only a small portion of the sources researched during the preparation of this book. Reference numbers appearing within or at the end of sentences refer, specifically, to that sentence's content, generally being a quotation or a disease incidence statistic. Those at the end of paragraphs refer more broadly to the subject matter within the preceding paragraph or paragraphs.

CDC and WHO prevalence and incidence data is cited by virtually all medical historians and researchers and I relied heavily on those two sources throughout the book. The Mayo Clinic, Cleveland Clinic, and Johns Hopkins references are included as authoritative sources of clinical information regarding disease presentation, diagnosis, progression, complications, and treatment. Similarly, the Merck Manual is written by recognized clinical experts and is a relied upon reference in the personal library of virtually every medical student and resident physician. Cited journal articles represent peer-reviewed research or subject reviews and are included for readers who wish a more detailed discussion of a particular aspect of the work summarized in the text.

Biographical profiles of prominent researchers and clinicians, written by the editors of the Encyclopedia Britannica and specialty museum curators, provide interesting historical background information. Lesser credentialed references and Internet videos were critically reviewed for accuracy before listing, and are included, like others, for their clarity and/or readability. Footnotes list supplemental reading, either historical novels or history books of potential interest to the reader.

All included pictures and figures are drawn from the public domain, based on elapsed time from initial publication or from U.S. government institutions (NIH, CDC, Smithsonian, etc.). All can be found in multiple web sites, with the particular Internet source selected for this book credited in the picture caption as well as the artist and original source, whenever applicable or known.

****

The book is divided into chapters, beginning with an introductory chapter outlining historical theories of disease causation, prevention, and cure, which is intended to provide some perspective and contextual understanding for the ensuing disease-specific chapters. Included chapters cover contagious diseases, vector-borne/zoonotic diseases, fecal-oral diseases, sexually transmitted diseases, substance use disorders, parasitic diseases, nutritional diseases, fungal diseases, and soil-related bacterial diseases of major historical impact afflicting Americans in the years predating the current era of disease identification, understanding, and treatment.

Contagious diseases are generally spread person-to-person by bacteria or viruses enveloped in respiration droplets, diffused into the air by an infected person during talking, sneezing, or coughing. Zoonotic diseases are spread from animals to humans by direct contact with the infected animal (or its bodily fluids), ingesting infected meat or animal-contaminated food or water, or by an intermediary vector ("vector-borne") such as mosquitoes, fleas, lice, and ticks.

Fecal-oral diseases are acquired by ingesting water or food contaminated by the feces of an infected individual. Commonly, drinking water is tainted by primitive (or non-existent) sewage systems and food by using human waste for fertilizer. An infected individual can unknowingly spread fecal-oral diseases by handling food or eating/cooking utensils without appropriate handwashing following a bowel movement.

Sexually transmitted diseases are communicated with the exchange of bodily fluids during sexual intercourse or by intimate contact with an open lesion (sore) associated with a particular disease. Substance use disorders are self-inflicted indulgences, often resulting in addictions. The two nutritional diseases discussed in the text are caused by inadequate dietary intake of an essential vitamin, specifically vitamins D and C.

Parasitic diseases are acquired through multiple modes including contact with fecally contaminated soil, insect vectors, ingestion of parasite contaminated food, and sexual intercourse. Fungal diseases are acquired by inhaling environmental fungal spores, contagious contact with infectious skin dermatophytes, or overgrowth of fungi normally inhabiting the skin or vagina. Soil-related bacterial infections are caused by soil contamination of open wounds, or by inhalation, ingestion, or skin contact with soil-indigenous bacterial spores.

Of note, the inclusion of a disease within a particular category is somewhat arbitrary in many cases. Malaria, for example, is listed as a vector-borne disease, which it clearly is. However, it is a parasite sporozoite that the vector mosquito carries from person-to-person, so it could reasonably be included within the parasitic disease category, as well. Similarly, anthrax is a soil-related bacterial disease, but is most commonly contracted by contact with an infected animal or animal parts so could, alternatively, be included in the zoonotic disease chapter.

Of additional note, dates regarding the introduction of vaccines and antibiotics can be very confusing. There is often a long time period—sometimes spanning decades—between the laboratory identification of a viable vaccine or antibiotic and its licensed approval for general use. I have tried to be specific with respect to the dates identified, but have been purposefully vague in some instances as widespread use frequently predated final licensure, much like the COVID-19 vaccines were in general use under "emergency use authorization" long before final FDA approval.

****

A recurring note of concern ends many of the disease sections throughout the text. The concern is the omnipresent threat of disease emergence or re-emergence in localized, epidemic or pandemic forms, potentially impacting the lives of many. The threat is very real and multifactorial, but centers on two principal areas of concern. The first is waning vaccine immunities in much of the world's population, including the U.S., coupled with the current trend of vaccine hesitancy. An unvaccinated or inadequately vaccinated populus is at grave risk, particularly in a global world where disease transmission from one area to the next is an ever-present possibility. Moreover, effective vaccines are not currently available for many diseases, representing a broad area of needed research and development.

The second concern is ever-increasing bacterial resistance to existing antibiotics. The emergence of "superbugs," resistant to multiple or all antibiotics, is almost a daily topic of headline news. Critics note the lack of new antibiotics to combat these organisms and the associated lack of research and development efforts and money to address this area of universal need.

Similarly, the emergence of insecticide resistant mosquitoes and other disease transmitting vectors has limited the ability of the World Health Organization (WHO) and other national and international health organizations to combat malaria and other vector-borne diseases. Climate change has lengthened the breading season and fostered the widespread dissemination of mosquitoes, ticks, and other insect vectors, further complicating international disease prevention efforts.[2] Additionally, the lack of monies committed by the global community for prevention and treatment of diseases has hampered many of the initiatives promoted by the WHO and other agencies.

Enjoy.

---

[2] The reader might find the article in *The Washington Post* (November 2, 2023) titled "Malaria's Deadly Reach is Growing" of interest. The article, written by Rachel Chason, Kevin Crowe, John Muyskens, and Jahi Chikwendiu, documents the alarming increase in malaria cases in Mozambique, attributed to climate change and the correspondingly longer breeding season for the *Anopheles* mosquito, principal transmitter of malaria between people.

Contents

About the Author

James A. Shaw is a recently retired academic orthopedic surgeon with more than 30 years of teaching, writing, and lecturing experience, accompanying an active clinical practice focused on hand surgery and joint replacement. He has published extensively in peer-reviewed journals, authored orthopedic textbook chapters, and has served on the review boards of several academic journals. He has been an invited speaker, moderator, and presentation commentator at many local, regional, and national/international orthopedic meetings.

Before entering medical school, Dr. Shaw received bachelor's and master's degrees in mechanical engineering from Cornell University and is the designer of two prosthetic knee replacements.

Dr. Shaw is an outdoor enthusiast, lover of travel, student of history, and a fan of historical novels. In addition to his ever-supporting wife, he is blessed with two wonderful daughters, both with PhDs in medically related fields, and three lively grandsons.

Chapter 1
Historical Theories of Disease Causation, Prevention, and Cure

Abstract An imbalance of vital humors (*yellow bile, black bile, phlegm, and blood*), first introduced by Hippocrates (460–370 BCE) and his followers in the fourth- and third-century BCE, remained the principal theory of disease causation well into the nineteenth century. Therapeutic corrections were focused on restoring humoral equilibrium through diet or purging—the latter achieved through bloodletting, emetics, diuretics, poultices, and laxatives. Diseases were felt to be acquired by inhaling foul-smelling air, referred to as the miasma theory of disease. Alcohol- and opioid-laced patent medicines flourished as "cure-alls" for virtually every type of disease.

The germ theory of disease, generally credited to the pioneering works of Louis Pasteur, Joseph Lister, and Robert Koch in the mid-1800s, reduced the understanding of disease to a simple interaction between a microorganism and host. Embraced more rapidly in Europe than America, antiseptic medical and surgical practices soon followed with a marked diminution of iatrogenic infections, as did more widespread attention to personal hygiene. Initially referred to as "non-filterable" disease-causing agents, viruses were definitively identified in the 1930s with the development of the electron microscope.

Vaccines were first introduced by English physician Edward Jenner in 1796 for the prevention of smallpox, followed over ensuing decades by vaccines for a large number of other diseases—many derived from killed or attenuated viruses. In 2020, modified messenger RNA vaccines were introduced, representing a new concept in vaccine development.

In 1909, the arsenic-based compound Salvarsan (arsphenamine) was introduced for the treatment of syphilis. Generally regarded as the first effective antimicrobial agent, Salvarsan was followed several decades later by sulfonamides, penicillin, and vast array of other antibiotics.

Current concerns referable to infectious diseases focus on ever-increasing microbial antibiotic resistance, waning vaccine immunities, vaccine hesitancy, and environmental changes favoring the propagation and spread of disease-transmitting insect vectors.

Without question, the earliest theories of disease were based on religious or demonic beliefs, linking the misfortunes of man to divine retribution for sins committed—a concept that continues to percolate through the minds of many, to date [1, 2].

Be that as it may, the first to consider that diseases had natural (vs. supernatural) causes was Hippocrates (460–370 BCE) and his followers in the fourth- and third-century BCE. Hippocrates postulated that disease was caused by an imbalance of four vital humors: *yellow bile, black bile, phlegm, and blood.* Illness was thought to occur when there was an excess or deficiency in one of the four humors, a theory that persisted for another 2000 years, well into the nineteenth century [3].

Hippocratic diagnoses were based on observations of a patient's excretions of sweat, urine, blood, vomitus, and stool. Therapeutic corrections of imbalance were focused on restoring equilibrium through diet or purging—the latter achieved through bloodletting, emetics, diuretics, poultices, and laxatives.

Seemingly barbaric and likely harmful from today's perspective, bloodletting was the principal tool in the armamentarium of physicians from the time of the ancient Greeks to the latter part of the nineteenth century. Considered the dominant humor, blood irregularities were felt to be responsible for most illnesses and releasing bad humors through bloodletting was the accepted standard of treatment for virtually all maladies [4, 5].

Bloodletting was performed as a systemic release of bad humors through venesection or arteriotomy or, alternatively, through localized release, by scarification and cupping or by application of leeches. Thumb lancets or pocketknife-like fleams were used to puncture superficial blood vessels, commonly the median cubital vein at the elbow, for a generalized release (Fig. 1.1). Suction cupping techniques or leeches were used to withdraw disease-causing humors from localized lesions such as an infected wound or the bubo of bubonic plague.

A likely example of an unknowing malfeasance was the bloodletting performed on former president George Washington (1732–1799). Following a wintry horseback ride, President Washington came down with a fulminant throat infection, possibly epiglottitis. He died within 24 h and during that time period he endured four

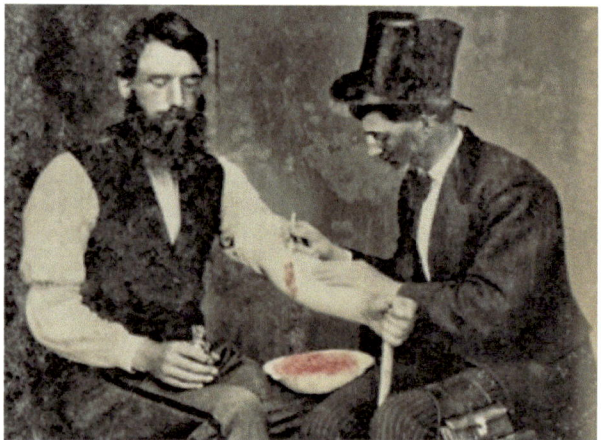

Fig. 1.1 Colorized photograph of bloodletting, Circa 1860. (Picture Source: https://en. wikipedia.org. The Burns Archive)

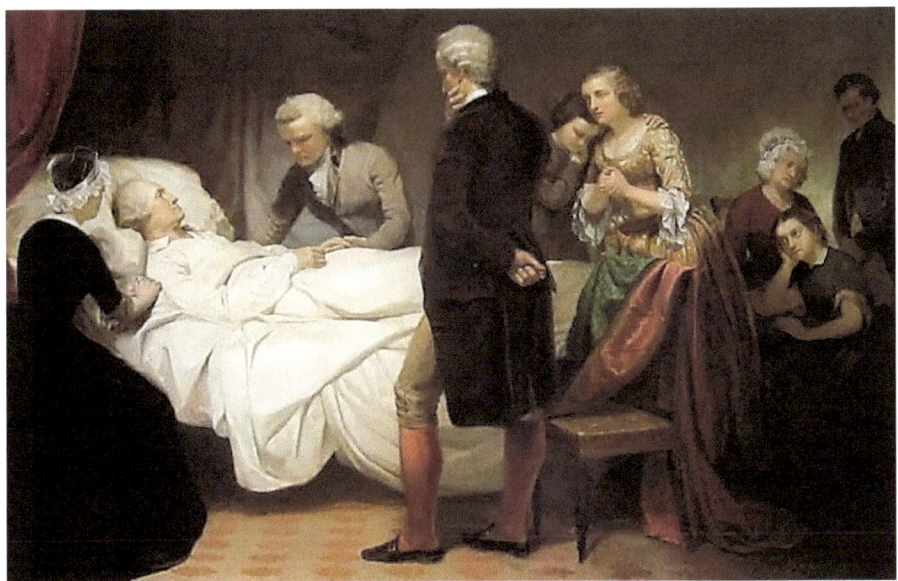

Fig. 1.2 Washington on his deathbed, circa 1851. Junius Brutus Stearns (1810–1885). (Picture Source: https://www.daytonartinstitute.org. Dayton Art Institute)

bloodlettings, amounting to 2500 ml or approximately 40% of his blood volume (Fig. 1.2). Although unlikely the direct cause of his death, it certainly was of no benefit [4, 6].

****

Evolving at some point in the Middle Ages, and persisting until the end of the nineteenth century, was the belief that the source of disease was *miasmas*. Simply put, malodorous vapors emanating from sewage-laden streets and waterways, swamps and wetlands, and putrefied body parts/lesions carried disease. Inhaling these smells caused illness. Emblematic of this concept is the origin of the name "malaria," which was derived from *mala aria*, Italian for "bad air" [7].

Arising from miasma theory were many ineffectual practices such as using smoky bonfires, burning incense, and wearing perfume to ward off diseases. Unwittingly, disease mitigation also benefited from miasma theory. Sewer systems were built, and swamps and wetlands drained to lessen miasmic smells, unknowingly eliminating the disease-causing bacteria which contaminated the drinking water and destroying the mosquito breeding grounds responsible for many vector-borne illnesses.

Although not understood from a modern perspective, the concept of disease contagion was well appreciated from the earliest of times—long before germ theory was first elucidated. In addition to miasmic transmission, early contagion theory suggested that diseases were spread by coming in direct contact with infected people, clothing, bedding, and food (all considered disease spreading *fomites*) and the most effective control of disease transmission was through quarantine of sick persons.

Early references to quarantine practices include the banishment and isolation of persons afflicted with leprosy (referred to as "unclean") during Biblical times, as depicted in the book of *Leviticus* [8]. Ships suspected of carrying plague were often quarantined offshore for 30–40 days during the Middle Ages, a waiting period known as *quarantinario* from the Italian word for 40 [9]. During the 1793 yellow fever epidemic in Philadelphia (then capital of the USA), federal government personnel isolated themselves by evacuating the city rather than risk contagious infection [9]. Early immigrants to America who were suspected of carrying transmissible diseases were often sent to quarantine from Ellis Island—a practice which continues to date under authority of the CDC's Division of Global Migration and Quarantine [10].

****

Germ theory revolutionized the practice of medicine, reducing the understanding of disease to a simple interaction between a microorganism and host. The French chemist and microbiologist Louis Pasteur, English surgeon Joseph Lister, and German physician Robert Koch are generally credited as the founding fathers of germ theory [11].

Louis Pasteur (1822–1895) is best known for his discoveries of microbial fermentation, pasteurization (which carries his name), and the foundational principles of vaccination. Based on a series of experiments on alcohol fermentation in the mid-1850s, Pasteur provided evidence that living organisms, not a series of inherent chemical reactions, caused the fermentation process. In 1865, he patented a method of heat sterilization to prevent spoilage of wine and other liquids. In milk, the process killed harmful bacteria, including the infective bovine tuberculosis organism, *Mycobacterium bovis*—representing a major advance in public health [12–14].

In related studies, Pasteur proposed that environmental microorganisms caused disease and infection, not an internal state of "humoral imbalance," or "spontaneously generated" microorganisms. Remarkably, he also discovered how to make vaccines from weakened/attenuated microorganisms, including the earliest vaccines against fowl cholera, anthrax, and rabies. In 1885, Pasteur and his colleagues successfully prevented a rabies infection in 9-year-old Joseph Meister, who had been bitten by a rabid dog, with a series of inactivated rabbit rabies virus inoculations [12–14].

Expanding on the work of Pasteur, Dr. Joseph Lister (1827–1912) postulated that environmental microorganisms colonized open (compound) fracture wounds, causing infection and sepsis. As a decontaminating germicide, he experimentally applied dilute carbolic acid to open wounds and surgical instruments, introduced weak carbolic acid hand washes for surgical staff, and used watery solutions of carbolic acid spray to reduce the level of germs in the air around the patient (Fig. 1.3). With the addition of these antiseptic adjuncts, infection rates in his practice decreased markedly. Feeling compelled to share the encouraging results of his clinical studies, he published two papers in *The Lancet* in 1867, outlining the technique [15, 16].

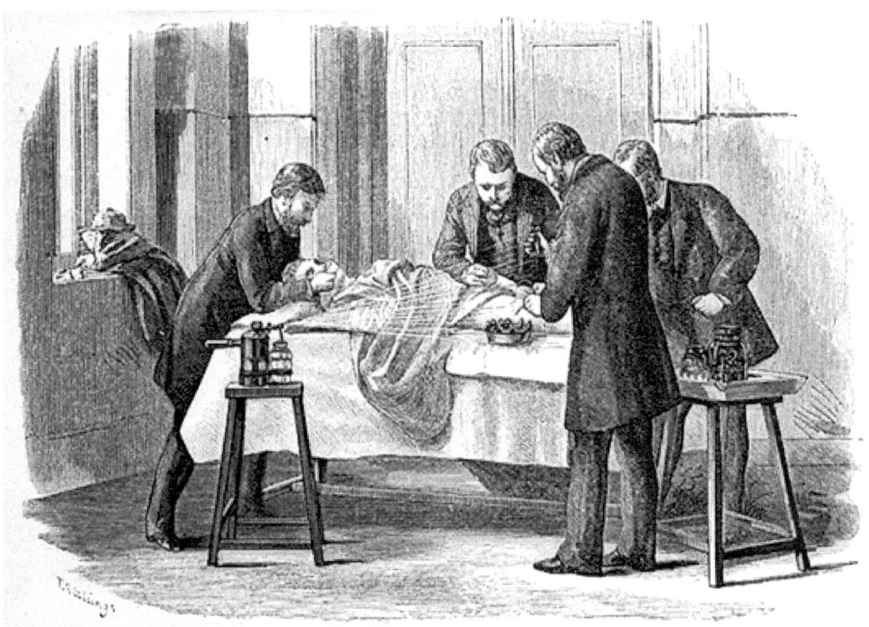

Fig. 1.3 Lister's antiseptic spray in use in an operating room, Circa 1882. (Picture Source: https://www.sciencemuseum.org.uk. *Antiseptic Surgery: Its Principles, Practice, History and Results* by W. Watson Cheyne. Wellcome Collection. Public Domain Mark)

Lister was the first to apply the science of germ theory to surgical practice. His antisepsis principles remain the basis of modern infection control and his revolutionary techniques made surgery much safer and helped to save countless lives.

Although germ theory was accepted relatively quickly in Europe, Lister's aseptic principles were met with cynicism and ignorance for many years in the USA. Bloodstained frocks and unwashed hands and instruments remained common well into the 1870s. Most notably, Dr. Willard Bliss and other attending physicians repeatedly probed President James A. Garfield's (1831–1881) gunshot wound over many weeks with unwashed fingers and instruments in unsuccessful attempts to retrieve the retained bullet after he was shot in an assassination attempt by Charles J. Guiteau on July 2, 1881.[1]

Garfield's gunshot wound was not immediately fatal, but he died of florid sepsis on 19 September 1881, 80 days after being shot. Autopsy findings showed no sign of infection around the retained bullet, itself, but active infection along the multiple soft-tissue tracks formed by probing unsterile fingers and instruments.

---

[1] The reader might find of interest *The Butchering Art: Joseph Lister's Quest to Transform the Grisly World of Victorian Medicine* (Scientific American/Farrar, Strauss, and Giroux, 2018) by Lindsey Fitzharris.

Subsequent to Garfield's death, Dr. Bliss was severely censured by the medical community for his blatant disregard of aseptic surgical techniques, which had by then become generally accepted principles of medical science and practice. Ridiculed in the press for his ineptitude, the phrase "Ignorance is Bliss" became part of the American lexicon [17].

During his trial, Guiteau argued that Garfield's death was due to medical malpractice, not his gunshot wound. The jury was not convinced and he was convicted of murder on January 5, 1882.

N.B.

Predating the works of Pasteur and Lister by several years—and one of the most historically under acknowledged advances in trauma management and sepsis mitigation—was the use of bromine as an antiseptic agent (antiputrefaction agent, as then appreciated) in the treatment of gangrenous wounds in the midst of the American Civil War [18].

Although infectious diseases (dysentery, typhoid fever, malaria, measles, etc.) were the principal causes of death during the Civil War, wound infections and sepsis following battlefield injuries took many thousands of lives as well. Faced with a staggering number of extremity wounds, largely caused by the bone-shattering/flesh-tearing impact of the 0.58 caliber Minié Ball, battlefield surgeons frequently opted for the expediency of amputations over attempts at limb salvage, which were then considered to be futile and infection-prone (Fig. 1.4).

Following his fortuitous observation that post-surgical infection rates were lower in recovery wards where bromine was used as a deodorizing spray, Dr. Middleton Goldsmith (1818–1887) began experimenting with bromine as a putrefaction/gangrene inhibitor during his service as a surgeon with the Army of the Cumberland.

In 1863 Goldsmith submitted a detailed report to the Surgeon General relaying his experimental observation that the application of bromine to gangrenous wounds decreased the mortality rate of patients under his care to under 3% from a generally reported average of over 40% [19]. Following his report, bromine antisepsis (anti-putrefaction) became a standard of care throughout Union military hospitals, with many lives saved.

Unfortunately, Goldsmith's experimental observations predated the elucidation of germ theory linking microbes to surgical infections. As such, he was unable to explain his clinical results in a scientifically rigorous fashion. That unfortunate fact, coupled with prideful post-war resistance from battle-savvy surgeons and physicians, delayed the acceptance of germ theory and the initiation of aseptic medical and surgical practices in the United States for many years after being acknowledged and routinely embraced in Europe—needlessly costing American lives to sepsis [19].

With respect to Dr. Goldsmith's legacy, bromine continued to be successfully used as a skin and wound antiseptic for many years following the war, but was largely supplanted over time by less tissue-toxic alternatives.

Fig. 1.4 Post-amputation patient with arm gangrene, Circa 1863. Edward Stauch. (Picture Source: https://www.civilwarmed. org. Medical and Surgical History of the War of the Rebellion, Surgical vol. 2, p. 739)

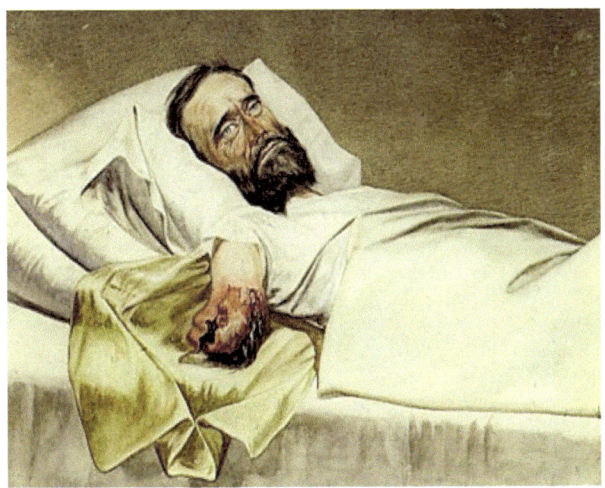

Robert Koch (1843–1910) is regarded as one of the founders of modern bacteriology, having correctly identified the causative organisms of anthrax (*Bacillus anthracis*), cholera (*Vibrio cholerae*), and tuberculosis (*Mycobacterium tuberculosis*), among others [20]. His seminal contribution to germ theory is his list of criteria necessary to establish a microorganism as a causative agent for a specific disease. Still applicable to date, and known as "Koch's postulates," the original criteria state [21]:

- The microorganism must be found in diseased, but not healthy individuals.
- The microorganism must be cultured from the diseased individual.
- Inoculation of a healthy individual [or animal] with the cultured microorganism must recapitulate the disease.
- The microorganism must be re-isolated from the inoculated, diseased individual and matched to the original microorganism.

N.B.
A positive aspect of the germ theory of disease was the introduction of soap and water to the lexicon of personal hygiene and sanitation. Simply put, most people stank through the mid-1800s until a causal link connecting personal cleanliness to disease was first established.

For many centuries preceding the Civil War, soap made from animal fat and ash lye had been used for cleaning clothes, but rarely for bathing. Early soaps were quite caustic to the skin and bathing was considered unhealthy (or immoral) by many. Tainted water was long associated with disease and body oils were felt to be protective. Perfumes were widely used to mask body odor.

With communicable diseases decimating combat troops during the Civil War, health officials began to encourage Union soldiers to wash with soap and water to remove bodily filth and what was then considered to be disease-causing odors (miasma). Concomitantly, nurses began to use soap to cleanse wounds to remove putrefactive smells. Seemingly helpful in stemming disease and infections on the battlefield, bathing for personal hygiene caught on with civilians, and demands for toilet soaps increased dramatically over ensuing years [22, 23].

As germ theory became more widely accepted in the States, health advocacy began encouraging bodily cleanliness. Ever-increasing social mores promoted sexy-smooth skin, silky hair and odor-free bodies. Social status and racial stereotypes were often used to advertise soap products (Fig. 1.5). Some ads depicted soaps as purveyors of social progress and universal morality. Personal cleanliness soon became tantamount to being a "good American" [23].

With the introduction of running water into many households (in addition to community bath houses in some locales) and the production and availability of less caustic soaps made from vegetable oils, cosmetic bathing became popular toward the end of the nineteenth century, particularly among the upper classes. Procter & Gamble introduced Ivory soap as one of the first perfumed products in 1879. Bestselling Palmolive soap was introduced in 1898 [24].

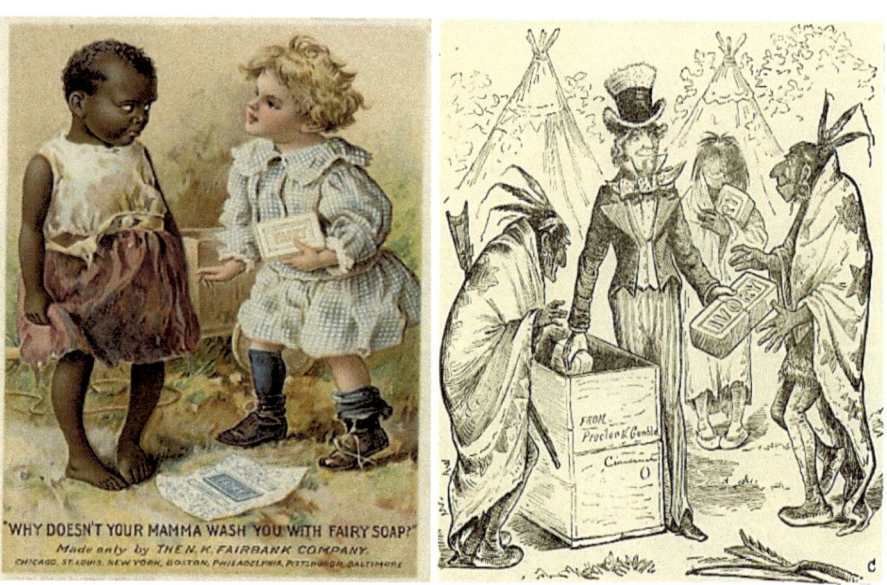

Fig. 1.5 Racial stereotype advertisements: Fairy Soap trade card, Circa 1900; Ivory Soap advertisement, Circa 1883. (Picture Source: https://www.si.edu. Smithsonian Institution)

Self-evidently, germ theory did not provide insight into the cause of many diseases, including those associated with malnutrition, cancers, aging, autoimmune disorders, obesity, etc. Furthermore, over time it became increasingly evident that disease causation was not always unifactorial, but a complex "web" of contributing factors including environmental and socio-economic influences [7].

****

While germ theory revolutionized the understanding of infectious diseases, it did not immediately lead to cures, awaiting the development of antibiotics in the 1940s. On the other hand, effective vaccines were first introduced long before bacteria were identified and even longer before the mysterious "filterable" (able to pass through a filter) disease agents, later called viruses, were readily isolated following the introduction of the electron microscope in 1931 [25].

With respect to a brief historical summary, major steps in vaccine development are noted below [26, 27], with more detailed discussions included within the text of the individual disease sections that follow.

- English physician Edward Jenner is credited with development of the first vaccine in 1796. Following the risky practice of variolation as an immunization technique for smallpox, Jenner expanded on the observation that persons who had recovered from the relatively mild disease of cowpox showed apparent immunity to smallpox. His experimentally proven vaccination technique involved transferring pus from an infected person's cowpox sore into superficial incisions made on the arms of healthy individuals. Referred to as "arm-to-arm" inoculation, persons generally developed a mild cowpox infection following the inoculation procedure and upon recovery benefited from its associated immunity to smallpox.
- In 1885, Louis Pasteur and his colleagues successfully prevented a rabies infection in a 9-year-old boy who had been bitten by a rabid dog, with a series of inactivated rabbit rabies virus inoculations.
- In 1890, Shibasaburo Kitasato developed a diphtheria antitoxin, derived from serum which was drawn from horses which had been inoculated with diphtheria toxin. Antibodies produced by the inoculated horses neutralized the diphtheria toxin, mitigating its toxic effects.
- In the early 1900s, vaccines were developed for pertussis, diphtheria, and tetanus and combined into the DTP vaccine in 1948.
- In 1945, the first influenza vaccine was approved for military use, followed by its approval for general civilian use in 1946.
- From 1952 to 1955, Dr. Jonas Salk developed the first polio vaccine, later supplanted by the easier to administer live-attenuated (oral) vaccine developed by Dr. Albert Sabin in 1960.
- Dr. Maurice Hillman developed the measles (1963), mumps (1967), and rubella (1969) vaccines while working at the Merck laboratories, later combined into the single shot MMR inoculation.
- In more recent history, vaccines against hepatitis, pneumococcal pneumonia, *Haemophilus influenzae*, human papillomavirus (HPV), shingles, meningococ-

cal meningitis, rotavirus, malaria, Ebola, and other diseases have been developed.

• In 2020, novel messenger RNA vaccines were introduced by Moderna and *Pfizer*-BioNTech to protect against infection with the coronavirus responsible for the COVID-19 pandemic.

****

Comparable to the inestimable importance of vaccines in preventing the spread of communicable diseases, the introduction of antibiotics into clinical use during the twentieth century was arguably one of the most important medical breakthroughs of all time and proved to be of enormous benefit in treating active infections and saving lives. When used prophylactically, antibiotics also proved to be helpful in controlling infectious outbreaks in areas of endemic communicable diseases and of critical importance in lessening the incidence of contaminating infections during surgical procedures [28].

N.B.
Sandwiched between the era of bloodletting and the era of antibiotics was the era of "Patent Medicines." During the eighteenth, nineteenth and early twentieth centuries, most Americans had little understanding of physiology, biochemistry or medicine. Physicians were not always knowledgeable, well trained, or of reputable standing and hospitals were often regarded as places to die [29].

Patent medicines (Fig. 1.6) provided a hopeful panacea when little else was available. The products were seldom actually patented, as the patent process would have required an exact listing of the ingredients, which generally consisted of proprietary combinations of herbs, vegetable extracts and sugar, blended together with generous amounts of alcohol, and commonly fortified with opium, morphine or cocaine. Most often, the medicines were simply trademarked [29, 30].

During the Mexican War and the Civil War communicable diseases spread rampantly, with two-thirds of soldiers dying of disease, not combat wounds. Patent medicines were promoted as cure-alls and unscrupulously distributed to needy troops by patent medicine manufacturers. On the home front, patent medicines were similarly marketed as cures for virtually every human ailment—from consumption to depression to rheumatism to digestive ailments to melancholy to gout to "women's problems" [29].

Like patent medicines, "patented" electrical devices of all shapes and sizes flourished in the 1800s, all purporting to cure whatever ailed you by administering a mild electrical shock, heat, or mechanical vibrations. Most were harmless, almost all were profitable, but none were truly useful or curative [31].

Fig. 1.6 Patent medicine advertisement, Circa 1881. (Picture Source: https:// exhibit.sos.ca.gov. California State Archives)

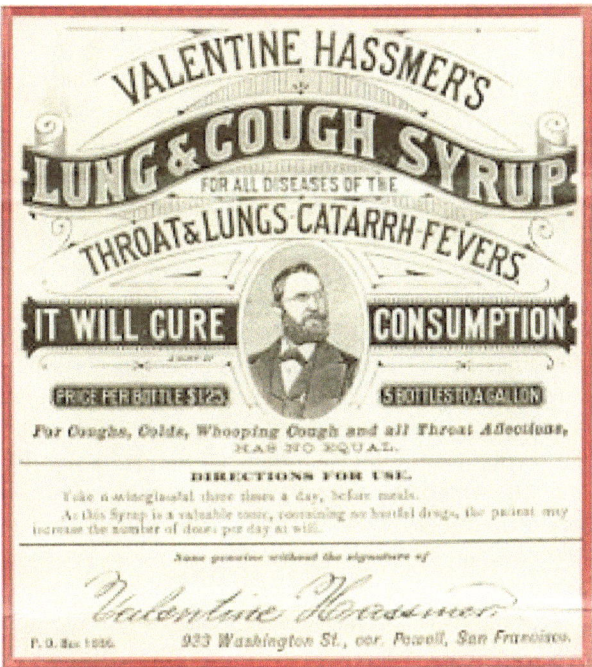

German physician Paul Ehrlich (1854–1915) and Scottish physician and microbiologist Alexander Fleming (1881–1955) are generally regarded as the founding fathers of the antibiotic era. In 1909, Ehrlich discovered that the arsenic-based compound Salvarsan (arsphenamine) was effective in the treatment of *Treponema pallidum*, the causative organism of syphilis. Used to treat syphilis until the 1940s, arsphenamine is generally regarded as the first modern antimicrobial agent.

Salvarsan was superseded by the sulfonamide drug Prontosil, developed in 1931 by Gerhard Domagk (1895–1964), a bacteriologist at the Bayer pharmaceutical company. Sulfonamides, all of which are related to the compound sulfanilamide, were the first successful broad-spectrum antimicrobials (which are still in use today), but proved limited in their application by the rapid development of bacterial resistance, and were largely supplanted by the subsequent discovery/development of penicillin [28, 32, 33].

Alexander Fleming is credited with the discovery of penicillin in 1928, although others, including Joseph Lister (1827–1912), likely preceded him [32]. Fleming accidentally observed the antimicrobial property of *Penicillium notatum* on *Staphylococcus* bacteria in his laboratory in 1928. The bread-derived *Penicillium* mold had inadvertently contaminated a Petri dish containing Staph organisms which he had unintentionally left uncovered while on holiday.

Fleming subsequently showed that the *Penicillium* mold inhibited bacterial growth at very low concentrations, but it took years before penicillin was successfully purified by scientists at Oxford University and could be economically manufactured on a large scale. By D-Day 1944, penicillin was available in sufficient quantity to treat infected war wounds and venereal diseases (syphilis and gonorrhea) in Allied troops. Referred to as a "wonder drug," it became commercially available for general use in 1945 [28, 32–35].

The ensuing 20 years is often referred to as the "Golden Age" of antibiotic discovery [28, 32]. Aminoglycosides (*Gentamicin*) were clinically introduced in 1946, tetracyclines (*Tetracycline*) in 1948, macrolides (*Erythromycin*) in 1952, glycopeptides (*Vancomycin*) in 1958, and cephalosporins (*Keflex*) in 1964, among many others [28].

However, since the 1970s few new antibiotics have been developed, with current clinical trials largely focused on derivatives of existing antibiotics or antibiotic combinations. This fact, coupled with the recent emergence of multidrug-resistant strains of bacteria, likely spurred by over/inappropriate use of antibiotics (e.g., for viral infections), patients not completing a full course of antibiotics and/or long-term administration of antibiotics for suppression of chronic infections—coupled with the remarkable adaptive capabilities of bacteria—now threatens the usefulness of these life-saving medications and has created a critical imperative for new research and development [28, 32–35].

In addition to ever-increasing antibiotic resistance, current concerns referable to infectious diseases focus on waning vaccine immunities, vaccine hesitancy, and environmental changes favoring the propagation and spread of disease-transmitting insect vectors.

References

1. de Wet CL. Is illness God's punishment? Theological perspectives from the Bible and the Apocrypha. Academic Research/LitNet Akademies; 2020. https://www.litnet.co.za.
2. Baden J, Moss C. Blaming Ebola on God's wrath is worse than you think. Slate. 2014. https://www.newscientist.com.
3. Lagay F. The legacy of humoral medicine. AMA J Ethics. 2002;4(7):206–8. https://journalofethics.ama-assn.org.
4. Greenstone G. The history of bloodletting. BCMJ. 2010;52(1):12–4. http://bcmj.org.
5. Nicola S. What to know about the history of bloodletting. WebMD; 2022. https://www.webmd.com.
6. Cheatham ML. The death of George Washington: an end to the controversy? Am Surg. 2008;74(8):770–4. https://pubmed.ncbi.nlm.nih.gov.
7. LaMorte WW. Historical views of causation. Boston University School of Public Health; 2019. https://sphweb.bumc.bu.edu.
8. Gensini GF, Yacoub MH, Conti AA. The concept of quarantine in history: from plague to SARS. J Infect. 2004;49(4):257–61. https://www.journalofinfection.com.
9. Klibanoff E. A history of quarantines, from bubonic plague to Typhoid Mary. NPR; 2020. https://npr.org.
10. CDC. History of quarantine. Centers for Disease Control and Prevention, National Center for Emerging and Zoonotic Infectious Diseases (NCEZID), Division of Global Migration and Quarantine (DGMQ); 2020. https://www.cdc.gov.
11. Curiosity Collections Harvard Library. Germ theory. Cambridge: Harvard University/Harvard Library; 2022. https://curiosity.lib.harvard.edu.

12. Science History Institute. Louis Pasteur. Science History Institute Museum and Library. Undated. https://sciencehistory.org.
13. Smith KA. Louis Pasteur, the father of immunology? Front Immunol. 2012;3:68. https://www.ncbi.nlm.nih.gov.
14. Liman A. Louis Pasteur. Encyclopedia Britannica, Inc.; 2023. https://www.britannica.com.
15. Pitt D, Aubin J-M. Joseph Lister: father of modern surgery. Can J Surg. 2012;55(5):8–9. https://www.ncbi.nlm.nih.gov.
16. Science Museum. Joseph Lister's antisepsis system. Science Museum; 2018. https://www.sciencemuseum.org.uk.
17. Herndon JH. Ignorance is bliss. Harvard Orthop J. 2013;15:74. https://www.orthojournalhms.org.
18. Trombold JM. Gangrene therapy and antisepsis before Lister: the Civil War contributions of Middleton Goldsmith of Louisville. Am Surg. 2011;77(9):11. https://pubned.ncbi.nlm.nih.gov.
19. Dalton K. The direct and logical consequence—germ theory and the Civil War. National Museum of Civil War Medicine; 2020. https://www.civilwarmed.org.
20. Lakhtakia R. The legacy of Robert Koch. Sultan Qaboos Univ Med J. 2014;14(1):37–41. https://www.ncbi.nlm.nih.gov.
21. Segre JA. What does it take to satisfy Koch's postulates two centuries later? Microbial genomics and *Propionibacterium acnes*. J Invest Dermatol. 2013;133(9):2141–2. https://www.ncbi.nlm.nih.gov.
22. Admin. Soap through the ages: the history and future of hygiene and soap. Launch My Beauty Product; 2020. https://launchmybeautyproduct.com.
23. Smithsonian. Bathing (body soaps and cleansers). Smithsonian Institution; Undated. https://www.si.edu.
24. Ridner J. The dirty history of soap. The Conversation; 2020. https://theconversation.com.
25. VacCoat. Electron microscope invention: a historical overview. VacCoat, Ltd.; 2023. https://vaccoat.com.
26. WHO. A brief history of vaccination. World Health Organization; 2023. https://www.who.int.
27. Saleh A, Qamar S, Tekin A, et al. Vaccine development throughout history. Cureus. 2012;13(7):e16635. https://www.ncbi.nlm.nih.gov.
28. Hutchings MI, Truman AW, Wilkinson B. Antibiotics: past, present and future. Curr Opin Microbiol. 2019;51:72–80. https://www.sciencedirect.com.
29. Bahnemann G. Quack cures and self-remedies: patent medicine. Digital Public Library of America; 2015. https://dp.la/exhibitions/patent-medicine/1860-1920.
30. Cock-Starkey C. The lure of laudanum, the Victorian's favorite drug. Mental Floss. 2023. https://www.mentalfloss.com.
31. Weber SN. Patent medicines to cure any ailment. California State Archives; 2023. https://www.sos.ca.gov.
32. Gould K. Antibiotics: from prehistory to the present day. J Antimicrob Chemother. 2016;71(3):572–5. https://academic.oup.com.
33. MyBiosource Editorial Team. A guide to the history of antibiotics. 2023. www.mybiosource.com.
34. Microbiology Society. The history of antibiotics. 2023. https://microbiologysociety.org.
35. Aminov RI. A brief history of the antibiotic era: lessons learned and challenges for the future. Front Microbiol. 2010;1:134. https://www.ncbi.nlm.nih.gov.

Chapter 2
Contagious Diseases

Abstract Contagious diseases are generally spread person-to-person by bacteria or viruses enveloped in respiration droplets, diffused into the air by an infected person during talking, sneezing, or coughing. Historically, some contagious diseases caused the deaths of millions, others caused widespread illnesses, and some frightening disfigurements or disabilities. A few have been relegated to the annals of history by massive vaccination campaigns and others are readily treated by antibiotics. However, some continue to inflict their wrath on wide segments of the global populus and others continue to infect vulnerable people who are unvaccinated or have waning vaccine immunities.

The contagious diseases discussed in this chapter, along with their historical names and monikers, are: 1918 Pandemic Influenza (*Spanish Flu, Three-Day Fever, Trench Fever, Blue Death*); Hansen's Disease (*Leprosy*); 1918 Pandemic Influenza (*Spanish Flu, Three-Day Fever, Trench Fever, Blue Death*); Hansen's Disease (*Leprosy*); Smallpox (*Pox, Red Plague, Speckled Monster*); Rubeola (*Measles*); Rubella (*German Measles, Three-Day Measles*); Tuberculosis (*Phthisis, White Death, Consumption*); Group A Streptococcal Disease (*Scarlet Fever, Scarlatina, Quincy*); Varicella (*Chickenpox*); Diphtheria (*Boulogne Sore Throat, "The Strangler of Children," Throat Distemper*); Pertussis (*Whooping Cough*); Mumps (*Parotitis*); Meningitis (*Spinal Meningitis*).

1918 Pandemic Influenza (*Spanish Flu, Three-Day Fever, Trench Fever, Blue Death*)

The 1918 influenza pandemic was the deadliest pandemic in modern history [1]. The pandemic killed an estimated 50 million people worldwide (some estimates double that figure), with about 675,000 deaths in the USA alone—referable to a population one-third the current census. An estimated one-third of the world's

J. A. Shaw, *Historical Diseases from a Modern Perspective*,
https://doi.org/10.1007/978-3-031-52346-5_2

population (approximately 500 million persons) were infected, with debilitating economic and social repercussions virtually everywhere. Crowded urban areas in the USA and throughout the world were the most adversely affected [1, 2].

The influenza pandemic began during the waning months of WWI, corresponding roughly to the time period of America's active involvement in the conflict. In parallel with the staggering civilian influenza mortality, WWI (1914–1918) claimed approximately 8,500,000 lives among Allied and Central Powers soldiers from a combination of war-related injuries and disease [3].

Specifically, the U.S. military suffered 116,516 deaths during WWI,[1] of which approximately 53,000 were combat-related [4] and around 45,000 influenza-related [5]—suggesting that equivalently lethal wars were being waged on and off the battlefield, principally against influenza. Troops from other Allied and Central Power nations were similarly affected, perhaps hastening the end to the war, but the U.S. military likely suffered the highest influenza morbidity with 26% of the army sickened—representing over one million men [5].

****

By laboratory sequencing of viral DNA from exhumed influenza victims, it is now known that the 1918 pandemic was caused by an H1N1 influenza virus, with genes of avian (H5N1) origin—work spearheaded by Dr. Jeffery Taubenberger at the Armed Forces Institute of Pathology (AFIP) and published in *Nature* in 2005 [6].

At the time of the 1918 pandemic, however, viruses were unknown as disease-causing agents, only discovered with the development of the electron microscope in the 1930s. Without the benefit of modern diagnostic tools, a common assumption was that the pandemic was caused by a bacillus bacterium ("Pfeiffer's bacillus," now known as *Haemophilus influenzae*), found in the lungs of some patients at autopsy [7]. Nevertheless, lacking uniform and consistent bacterial evidence, many other etiology theories were advanced, including the hypothesis that the pandemic was caused by an unknown biologic agent introduced by the Germans as a weapon of war.

The origin of the 1918 pandemic remains a source of debate. Some subscribe to an Asian origin. Others suggest that the pandemic sprung from the trenches of WWI ("trench fever") or congested troop hospitals or training camps in Europe or the USA. The Allied hospital camp in Étaples, France, and Camp Funston, a U.S. Army training camp located on Fort Riley, southwest of Manhattan, Kansas, are commonly cited niduses of possible origin [5]. Other evidence implicates the nearby farming community of Haskell County, Kansas, where several early cases were identified and where migratory birds, pigs, and humans were intermixed, offering a plausible originating chain of transmission from animals to humans [8]. Whatever the origin, severe crowding of troops in hospital camps, training camps, holding areas, and on transport ships and trains created breeding grounds of contagion.

---

[1]Mortality data as reported by the U.S. War Department in February 1924. U.S. casualties as amended by the Statistical Services Center, Office of the Secretary of Defense, Nov. 7, 1957 [3].

Without question, the movement of troops around the globe fostered worldwide dissemination.

There were three recognized peaks or waves in the 1918 pandemic during its 15-month duration [2, 9], much like those which occurred during the COVID-19 pandemic. In March of 1918, more than 100 cases were reported at Camp Funston in Fort Riley, Kansas, soon followed by many hundreds more. Being the first recognized outbreak in America, the camp is considered by some epidemiologists as the origin of the worldwide pandemic, as noted above.

The initial wave following the Camp Funston outbreak was relatively mild, causing comparatively few deaths. However, the pandemic peaked in a second more virulent wave in the fall of 1918, causing most of the deaths in the USA and throughout the world (Fig. 2.1). A third peak occurred in the winter and spring of 1919, largely self-extinguishing during the summer and fall of 1919, but also responsible for considerable mortality. Persistent cases did linger into 1920, however, accounting for an "unofficial" fourth wave in the minds of some epidemiologists.

For a majority of people, the symptoms of the 1918 flu were similar to current flu strains: fever and chills, cough, headache, body aches, sore throat, loss of appetite, runny nose, and fatigue. The nickname "three-day fever" is credited to Colonel Sottau of the Army Medical Service when he observed that the typical infection course was 3 days' incubation, 3 days' fever, and 3 days' convalescence [10]. Unfortunately, many did not fare so well. Bacterial pneumonia was a frequent secondary complication. Without the benefit of antibiotics, death often followed (Fig. 2.2).

However, the unique and frightening feature of the 1918 pandemic was the high mortality rate in young healthy adults, age 20–40 years [2]. The affected patients' lungs rapidly filled with a thick exudate creating an agonizing "air hunger," their bodies starved of oxygen in a literal state of suffocation. Without the benefit of mechanical respirators, the resultant heliotrope cyanosis (a bluish coloration of the skin and extremities) was a sure sign of impending death—frequently occurring

Fig. 2.1 Emergency hospital at Camp Funston, Kansas, 1918. (Picture Source: https://www.smithsonianmag.com)

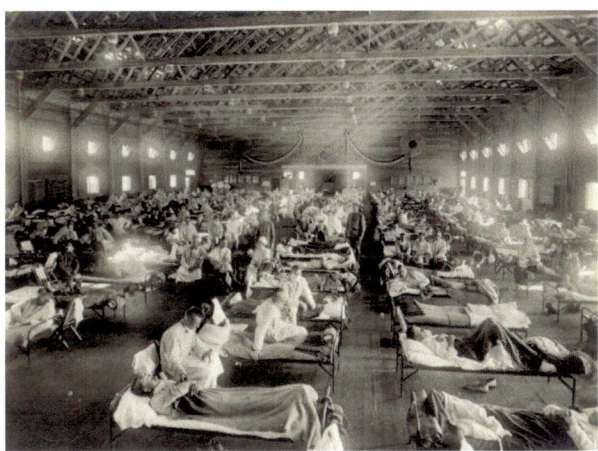

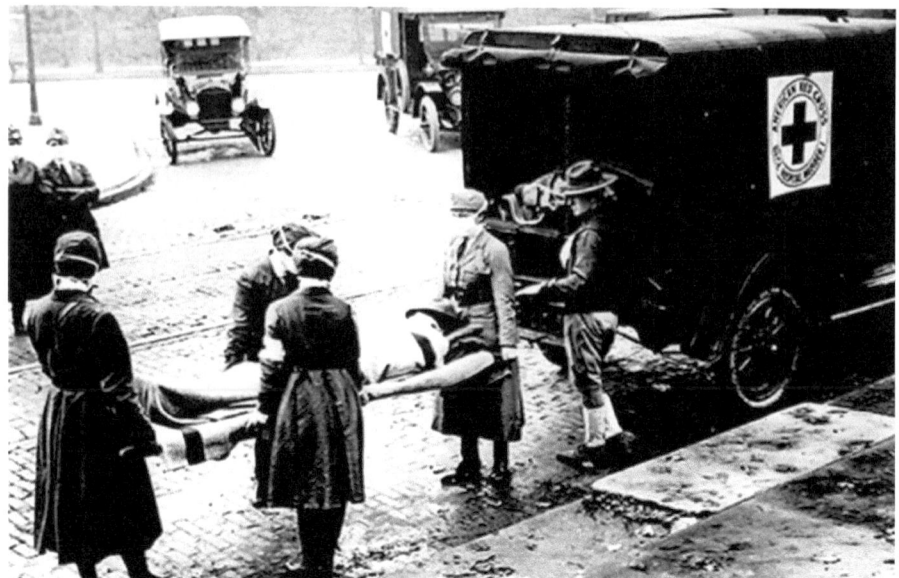

Fig. 2.2 Transport of an influenza patient, 1918. (Picture Source: https://www.cdc.gov. CDC)

within hours of the onset of symptoms—and the source of the infamous moniker "blue death." The pathophysiology of this severe inflammatory response is likely a form of cytokine storm, possibly similar to that experienced by some patients with COVID-19 infections [11].

With no vaccines available, no antiviral drugs, no intravenous monoclonal antibody therapies, no steroids or other anti-inflammatory drugs, and no mechanical respirators, patients were totally dependent on their own immune systems to combat the disease. In many cases that was sufficient, in many others it was not.

Non-pharmaceutical protocols were instituted to help control the spread of disease. Citizens were ordered to wear masks, schools, theaters, and businesses were shut down, and good personal hygiene and disinfectant use were encouraged. Despite these best-intentioned modalities, bodies piled up in makeshift morgues throughout the country and, out of necessity, were frequently disposed of in mass graves before the virus ended its global parade of death.

The term "Spanish Flu" is the most commonly used name for 1918 pandemic influenza. Interestingly, the name has no bearing referable to the pandemic's true origin or pathology but stems from politics, pure and simple. Self-evidently, the 1918 influenza outbreak affected troop strengths and preparedness on both sides of the WWI conflict—training camps, staging areas, transport ships, and battle-front trenches being principal foci of disease. Commanding generals and political leaders were reluctant to even acknowledge the pandemic, let alone reveal the number of troops affected, for fear of revealing a military disadvantage to the opposing side. Bad news was censored in an effort to maintain a positive home-front morale. As a propaganda tool, both sides blamed the other as originators of the pandemic [12].

During WWI, Spain was a neutral country with a free and uncensored press. Unlike many other countries, Spain's coverage of the pandemic was relatively forthright, with the first newspaper acknowledgement of an influenza outbreak in Madrid in May 1918. Subsequent reporting of widespread infections (including King Alfonso XIII) and mounting deaths went uncensored as well, creating a false impression that Spain was uniquely hard hit by the flu. Spain blamed France for transmission of the disease but the rest of the world latched on to Spain as the source of the pandemic. Although it is now generally agreed that Spain was not the epicenter of the disease, the term "Spanish Flu" has become a permanent part of our lexicon [12].

****

Seasonal influenza remains an ever-present disease burden in the USA and throughout the world. During the COVID-19 pandemic, the number of influenza infections remained relatively low compared to prior years, probably due to the populus observing isolation recommendations and wearing masks when in public. During the 2021–2022 influenza season, the CDC estimated that influenza was associated with 9 million illnesses, 4 million medical visits, 10,000 hospitalizations, and 5000 deaths, similar to the 2011–2012 disease burden [13].

More currently (October 1, 2022 through April 30, 2023), the CDC estimates that there were 27–54 million illnesses, 12–26 million medical visits, 300,000–650,000 hospitalizations, and 19,000–58,000 deaths in the USA from seasonal influenza—representing a significant increase in the number of cases compared to the previous year [13].

Hansen's Disease (*Leprosy*)

Few diseases conjure up the visceral horror of Hansen's disease, better known as leprosy. In advanced stages, the disease can be extremely disfiguring with nodular lesions (Fig. 2.3) on the skin (lepromas), non-healing ulcers on the feet, loss of eyebrows, nose disfigurement, resorption of toes and fingers, and paralysis of hands and feet, among other characteristic lesions.[2]

The scourge of humanity since antiquity, leprosy was historically regarded as a curse of God, associated with sin [14, 15]. With fear of contagion and pervasive social stigmatization, victims were routinely isolated, ostracized by family and community, treated inhumanely, and deprived of civil liberties.

Two closely related organisms are now known to cause leprosy, referred collectively as the *Mycobacterium leprae* complex [16]. The first, *Mycobacterium leprae*, was discovered by the Norwegian physician Dr. Gerhard Armauer Hansen in 1874

---

[2] The reader is referred to the World Health Organization's website for pictorial examples of leprosy disfigurement: https://photos.hq.who.int/galleries/227.

Fig. 2.3 Man with
leprosy. (Picture Source:
https://en.wikipedia.org.
From: Norman Purvis
Walker, *An Introduction to
Dermatology,* William
Hood & Co. 1905)

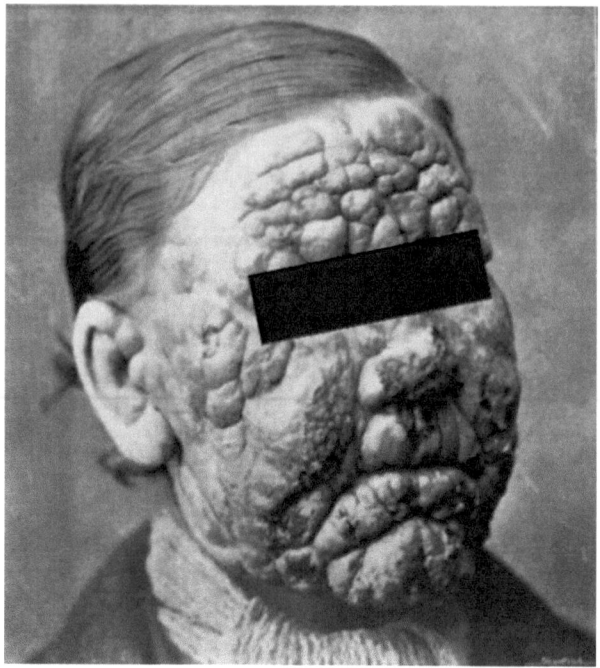

when searching for causal organisms in the skin lesions of leprosy patients—fostering the current terminology, "Hansen's disease." The second organism, the closely related *Mycobacterium lepromatosis*, was identified in Mexico in 2008 [16]. Neither organism can be cultured, lacking appropriate gene sequences to grow in a culture medium outside their human hosts. As such, a definitive diagnosis of infection is made by biopsy of characteristic skin lesions and direct microscopic identification of the infecting organism.

Contrary to popular belief, leprosy is not highly contagious and rarely causes death [16]. The only known reservoir of disease other than humans is the armadillo, representing a potential source of disease transmission [16, 17]. Most cases are thought to be transmitted from person-to-person via droplets from the nose and mouth during frequent and close contact with an infected and untreated individual [18]. Even after close contact, most immunocompetent people do not develop leprosy. Those that do are thought to have a poorly defined genetic predisposition, most healthy individuals having a natural immunity [16].

The *Mycobacterium leprae* bacteria multiplies very slowly. With an incubation period lasting an average of 5 years, symptoms may not occur for many years (1–20, or more) following infection, typically affecting the skin, peripheral nerves, limbs, nose, and eyes [18]. Historically, progressive disfigurement caused persons with leprosy to be feared and shunned by others, as noted above.

Beginning with the introduction of dapsone and other sulfones in the 1940s, leprosy could be successfully treated with antibiotics [16, 18]. Because of emerging antibiotic resistance in the 1960s, long-term multidrug regimens including rifampin and clofazimine are now generally used in conjunction with dapsone. Occasionally, lifelong suppressive antibiotics are required. Although leprosy is no longer contagious once antibiotics are initiated, antibiotics do not reverse any pre-existing nerve damage or deformity.

According to the January 2022 World Health Organization (WHO) website [18], more than 16 million patients have been treated free of cost with multidrug therapy (MTD) over the past 20 years, with a gradual reduction of new cases in several countries. In 2020, there were 127,558 new leprosy cases detected globally. Currently, leprosy medical care is carried out almost exclusively in outpatient clinics [18].

For lack of an available alternative, and based in logic on the similarities of their pathogenic bacteria, the tuberculosis Bacillus Calmette Guerin (BCG) vaccine is also used as a leprosy vaccine at this time. Clinical and observational studies suggest a protective efficacy of 26–61% in adults [19]. Organism-specific leprosy vaccines are currently under development and undergoing phase-1 clinical trials [19, 20].

The term "leper" is now considered a pejorative label, fostering hurtful discrimination and stigma against those afflicted with Hansen's disease. Leprosy Mission International suggests the term "person affected by leprosy" be used in its stead [15].

****

While relatively rare in America, 150–250 new cases of Hansen's disease are still reported each year in the USA, according to the CDC [21]. Most are in individuals who have emigrated from areas of the world where the disease is more common. Other cases appear to be contagiously acquired from handling infected armadillos [22]. Genetic mapping of population migrations over time suggests that leprosy was not present in the New World before Columbus arrived in the Americas but was introduced by Europeans and Africans during the early colonization period [22].

A leprosarium was established on the remote Hawaiian island of Molokai in 1866. Named Kalaupapa, the leprosy colony housed almost 8000 patients over 150 years of continuous operation, all of whom were taken from their families and homes and forced into a lifelong sentence of isolation.

Mandatory quarantine laws were abolished at Kalaupapa in 1969, a decade after Hawaii became a state and more than two decades after a cure with antibiotics was well established. Some patients chose to leave Molokai Island and reunite with their families. A few chose to remain, knowing no other life than one of forced isolation and state-supported welfare [23].

A leprosy hospital was established on Penikese Island off the southern coast of Massachusetts in 1904 to isolate and treat the state's patients with Hansen's disease. When opened, the Penikese hospital had five patients. After 16 years of operation, the remaining thirteen patients were transferred in sealed rail cars to the newly established federal leprosy hospital in Carville, Louisiana (Fig. 2.4) [24].

In 1921, the United States Public Health Service (USPHS) took over operation of Louisiana's 1894 Carville facility, becoming the National Leprosarium of the United States [25, 26]. Housing 400 patients at its peak, the facility gradually

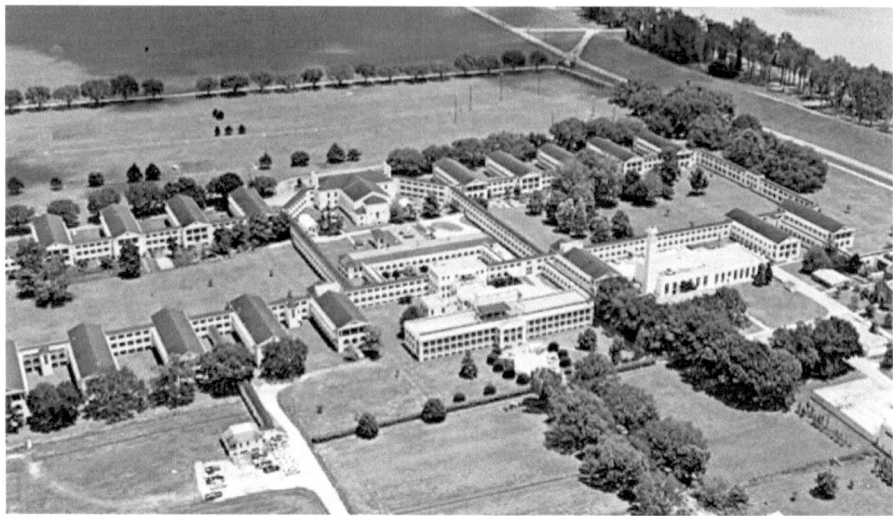

Fig. 2.4 The National Leprosarium at Carville. (Picture Source: https://prcno.org/revisiting-louisianas-medical-legacy-national-leprosarium-carville/. Louisiana Division of Historic Preservation)

transitioned from a "prison" of forced isolation to a facility on the forefront of medical research and humanitarian care.[3]

In the 1940s, Dr. Guy Henry Faget pioneered the use of sulfones to treat leprosy at Carville [25]. Replacing the largely ineffectual chaulmoogra and hydnocarpus oils, now of only historical interest [27], these antibiotics halted the progression and contagion of the disease, completely transforming the lives of patients with Hansen's disease.

Following antibiotic treatment and sequential negative skin biopsies, patients were allowed to leave the facility and resume normal lives. However, fearing continued hurtful stigmata, lacking employable skills, and knowing no other life than the one of isolation at Carville, some patients opted to stay, much like those at Kalaupapa.

In 1999, the few remaining patients were given a choice of a lifetime medical stipend, remaining on-site as an ambulatory care patient, or moving to the relocated leprosy hospital in Baton Rouge. In 2005, the Daughters of Charity, who ran the facility since its inception, officially ended their mission to care for patients at Carville. Today the facility is open as a museum [28].

---

[3] The reader is referred to Betty Martin's autobiography, *Miracle at Carvel*, (Doubleday & Co, 1950) and/or the historical novel, *The Second Life of Mirielle West*, by Amanda Skenandore (Kensington Publishing Corps., 2021) for depictions of life and treatment at Carville as a patient with leprosy.

Smallpox (*Pox, Red Plague, Speckled Monster*)

Smallpox was one of the deadliest and most contagious diseases to afflict mankind. Having killed hundreds of millions of people in the twentieth century alone [29, 30], the disease is now relegated to the annals of history, having been declared eradicated in 1980 by the World Health Organization (WHO) following a worldwide vaccination campaign—perhaps the most successful collaborative public health initiative in history [31]. The last known case was recorded in 1977 and the last outbreak in the USA occurred in 1949 [32].

A disease of ancient origin [31, 33], smallpox is caused by the variola virus, a member of the *Orthopoxvirus* genus. A nasty disease with no known cure and afflicting only humans, smallpox killed approximately 30% of those infected (with variola major) and often left survivors with deep pitted scars (pockmarks) for life. Some were rendered blind or infertile [31, 32].

Following an incubation period of 7–19 days, smallpox generally progressed with flu-like symptoms including high fever, body aches, prostration, and occasionally vomiting. Lasting several days, this early symptomatic period was followed by a highly contagious phase, identified by the formation of a characteristic rash—starting as small red spots on the tongue and mouth, followed by pustular lesions over the face and body (Fig. 2.5). If the infected person survived, the skin lesions scabbed over, leaving readily identifiable scars in most cases. Recovery afforded lifelong immunity, independent of the disease's severity [32].

Transmission of smallpox among people occurred principally during the highly contagious early-rash stage of the disease, when sores appeared in the mouth and throat. Close face-to-face contact communicated virus-laden droplets during a cough or sneeze. The pustular skin lesions also contained active virus particles, which could spread through contaminated bedding or clothing via hand-to-nose/mouth transfer. In enclosed spaces, aerosolized viruses circulating through the air were also a possible (albeit rare) mode of transmission. No evidence suggests that insect or animal vectors spread the disease [32].

Fig. 2.5 Smallpox victim showing characteristic skin lesions. (Picture Source: https://medicalmuseum. health.mil. National Museum of Health and Medicine. AFIP: Image 48135)

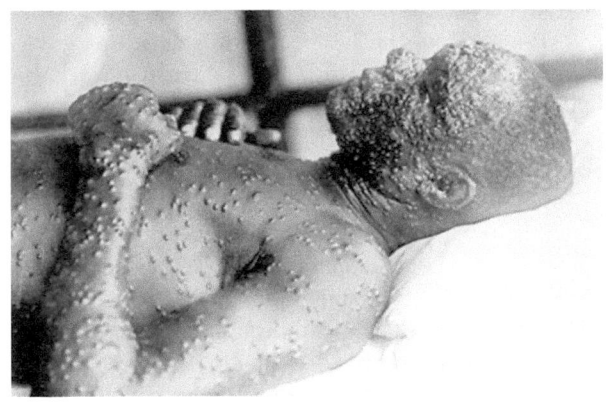

****

The origin of smallpox is unknown, but the existence of smallpox-like lesions on Egyptian mummies dates the history of known contagion to around 1000 BCE [33, 34]. With little doubt, the growth of civilizations, expanding trade routes, and global exploration spread the disease [34]. During the sixteenth century, European colonialism and African slave trade imported smallpox into the Caribbean and Central and South America. In the seventeenth century, European settlers brought smallpox to North America. With no prior exposure, Native Americans in both North and South America were decimated by smallpox and other European diseases, reducing indigenous populations by up to 90%, by some estimates [35]. Early American history was indelibly impacted by smallpox outbreaks within the colonies and by the parallel history of smallpox inoculations and vaccinations. Repeated outbreaks in Boston during the 1700s were particularly severe and among the best documented. During the smallpox epidemic of 1721, for example, approximately 840 Bostonians died, representing almost 8% of the city's population. Other notable outbreaks occurred in 1752, 1764, and 1775 [36].

Combating smallpox centered on two modern-day principles: isolation/quarantine and inoculation (variolation). During epidemics, Bostonians were required to prominently display warning signs of contagion within their households and remain isolated until resolution of symptoms. They were also encouraged to undergo prophylactic inoculations—all in an effort to contain the spread of disease [36].

Having learned about the West African practice of variolation from his slave, Onesimus, the Puritan minister Cotton Mather canvassed for its prophylactic use, most notably in response to the 1721 outbreak of smallpox in Boston. The variolation process involved extracting pus from the skin lesions of a mildly infected person and wiping the pus into superficial skin incisions made on the arm or leg of the person to be inoculated [36].

During the 1721–1722 epidemic, Mather convinced Dr. Zabdiel Boylston to inoculate Bostonians on an experimental basis. Following an uneventful trial inoculation of his 6-year-old son and two of his slaves, Boylston subsequently inoculated 282 patients, 6 of whom died (2%). Comparatively, of 5759 naturally acquired infections, 844 died (14.6%), cementing Dr. Boylston's heritage as the first person to introduce a successful inoculation to the practice of medicine in America [37, 38].

Despite Boylston's success, resistance to the variolation procedure was high among the citizens of Boston [36]. Controversial arguments ranged from its being a violation of "God's will," to the realization that patients suffered smallpox symptoms (although generally mild in comparison to native infections), occasionally died, and were actively contagious until fully recovered and thus required quarantine.

Be that as it may, the unassailable fact was that the procedure significantly lowered the risk of death from smallpox and was used successfully during subsequent epidemics in Philadelphia (1735) and Charleston (1738), among others [38]. Endorsement by Benjamin Franklin (whose son died of smallpox), John Adams and Thomas Jefferson, among others, helped assuage resistance to the procedure.

Debilitating outbreaks of smallpox among American troops during the siege of Boston and the siege of Quebec at the beginning of Revolutionary War prompted General George Washington (who had acquired a natural immunity following an

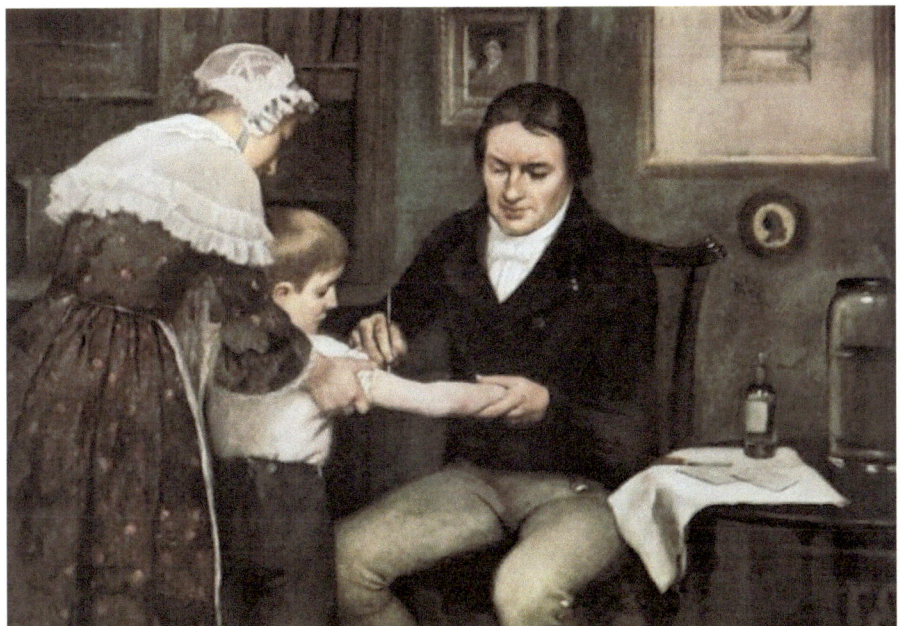

Fig. 2.6 Dr. Jenner performing his first vaccination. Circa 1910. Ernest Board. (Picture Source: https://en.Wikipedia.org/images.wellcome.ac.uk)

infection in the Caribbean) to order variolation on all new recruits and all those encamped at Valley Forge who did not have a natural immunity. This secretive and eminently successful initiative began in the spring of 1777 and continued through the following winter and is thought by many to have contributed significantly to the ultimate prevail of the Continental Army, without which the army may have irrevocably disintegrated due to disease[4] [39, 40].

A giant leap forward toward the elimination of the smallpox scourge occurred on May 17, 1796, when Dr. Edward Jenner (1749–1823) performed the world's first vaccination in Gloucestershire England (Fig. 2.6). Intrigued by local lore which purported that people who had recovered from cowpox infections were protected from the much more debilitating and lethal smallpox, Dr. Jenner inoculated 8-year-old James Phillips with pus obtained from a cowpox sore harvested from the hand of a local milkmaid, Sarah Nelmes. Two months after his uneventful recovery from his inoculation-induced cowpox infection, Philips was re-inoculated with pus from a human smallpox sore to test his acquired resistance to the disease. Young Phillips remained in perfect health, becoming the first person to receive a successful vaccination [31, 41].

Jenner's vaccination technique was not without difficulties. Cowpox did not occur widely, restricting the supply of cow-derived inoculum and necessitating the

---

[4]The reader might find *The Contagion of Liberty: The Politics of Smallpox in the American Revolution* (Hopkins University Press, Baltimore, MD, 2022) by Andrew M. Wehrman of interest.

formation of "arm-to-arm" vaccination clinics where cowpox inoculum was obtained directly from the pustules of humans who had contracted the disease and transferred to waiting patients. (Jenner later developed techniques where the inoculum could be dried and remotely transported, greatly facilitating the vaccination process.) Vaccination samples occasionally became contaminated with smallpox through unhygienic handling, creating public alarm. Heat instability made the inoculum less effective in warm climates, and unfounded rumors circulated that cowpox vaccination (Fig. 2.7) could turn people into cows [31, 41].

Nevertheless, through rigorous scientific testing Jenner's "vaccine inoculation" technique—later shortened to "vaccination" after the Latin for cow (*vacca*)—was definitively shown to protect against smallpox by 1801 [31]. In western regions of Europe and in the USA, variolation was outlawed and vaccination became compulsory during the mid-1800s. Concomitantly, vaccination certificates were required for international travel by some countries. Of obvious advantage over variolation, persons were not contagious following vaccination inoculations, as cowpox is not a communicable disease among humans. Moreover, cowpox seldom left a residual rash, only caused mild illness in most instances, and was rarely fatal [29, 31].

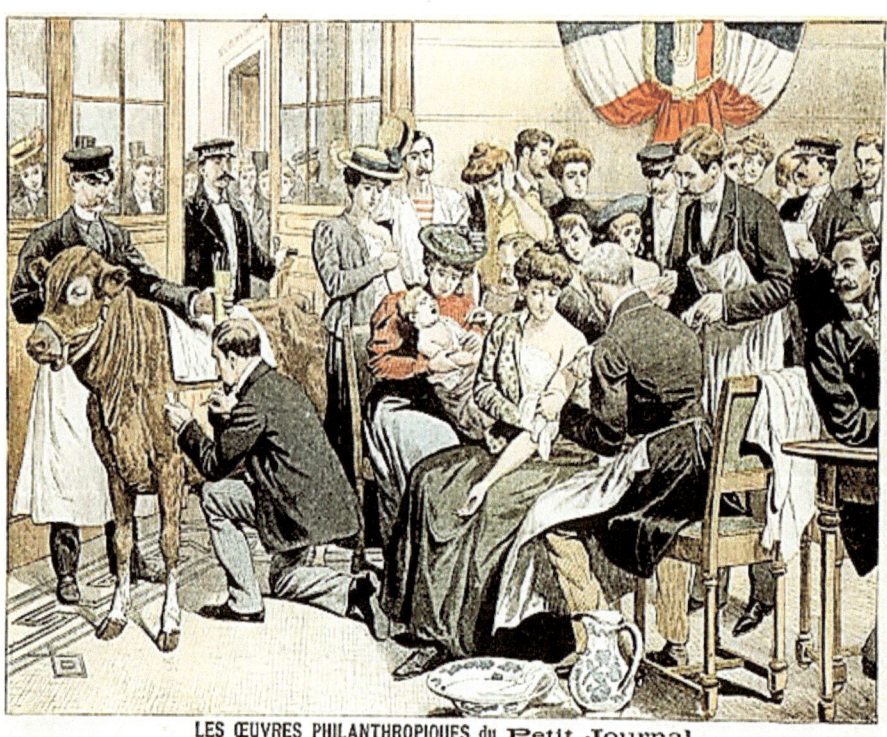

LES ŒUVRES PHILANTHROPIQUES du Petit Journal
La vaccination gratuite contre la variole dans le grand hall du Petit Journal

Fig. 2.7 French cowpox vaccination clinic, Paris. Circa 1905. (Picture Source: https://www.gettyimages.com. *Le Petit Journal*)

Despite the obvious public health imperative to rid the biosphere of smallpox and the overwhelming personal health advantage, vaccine skepticism persisted. To counter negative sentiment, extensive public information campaigns were instituted throughout the world, including the use of the iconic photograph of two boys—one vaccinated and one not—taken by Dr. Allan Warner at the Leicester Isolation Hospital in Leicester England, in 1901 (Fig. 2.8) [42].

While some European regions were able to eliminate smallpox by 1900, over 2 million persons continued to die each year, principally in third-world countries [31]. With the development of a heat-stable, freeze-dried vaccine made from the vaccinia virus (a poxvirus similar to smallpox, but less harmful), coupled with an increased worldwide solidarity in the campaign against the disease, smallpox was eliminated in western Europe, North America, and Japan in the 1950s [31].

The introduction of a bifurcated needle in the 1960s greatly facilitated the administration and appropriate dosing of vaccines (Fig. 2.9). This advance, in association

Fig. 2.8 Iconic image of two boys—one vaccinated, one not. Circa 1901. (Picture Source: https://www.nzherald.co.nz. Dr. Jenner's House)

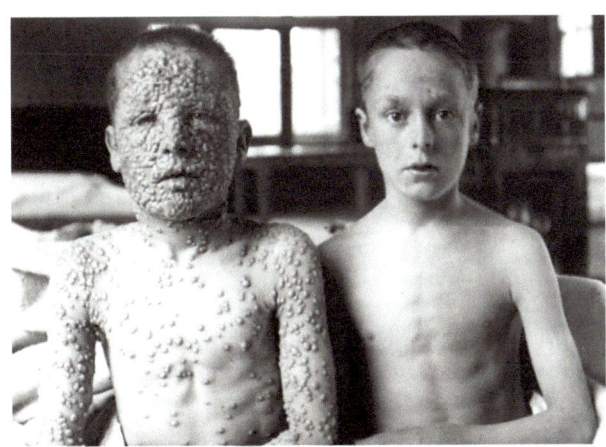

Fig. 2.9 The bifurcated needle used to administer smallpox vaccine. (Picture Source: https://en.wikipedia.org. CDC: Public Health Image Library)

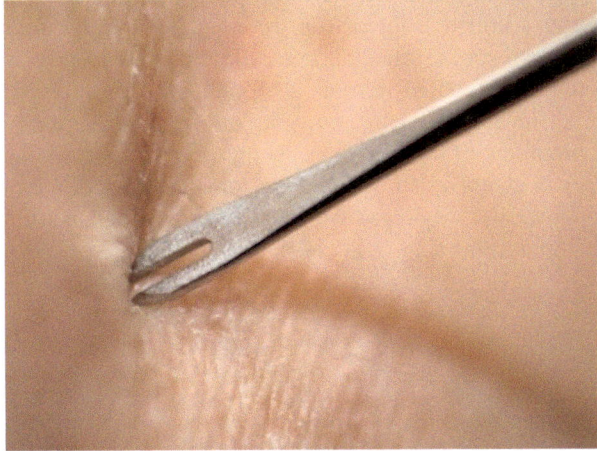

with the 1967 launch of the WHO's *Intensified Smallpox Eradication Program*, and the unprecedented multi-nation cooperative effort with respect to vaccine production, financing and volunteerism—all in the midst of the cold war!—defeated the global scourge and allowed the WHO to declare on May 8, 1980, that smallpox had been eliminated [31].

Routine smallpox vaccination is no longer recommended by the CDC as there have been no recorded cases of the disease since 1977.[5] Live-virus samples are stored in guarded laboratories at the CDC in Atlanta, Georgia, and the VECTOR Institute in Koltsovo, Russia, for research purposes only [34]. To protect against the remote chance of smallpox reemergence in an unvaccinated population and the possible use of the smallpox virus as an instrument of bioterrorism, the CDC maintains sufficient doses of vaccine in the *Strategic National Stockpile* for all U.S. citizens [43]. The current smallpox vaccine licensed in the USA is a lyophilized (freeze-dried), live-virus preparation of vaccinia virus and does not contain smallpox (variola) virus [45].

Rubeola (*Measles*)

Prior to the development of an effective vaccine in 1963, measles was a nearly ubiquitous disease of childhood. Highly contagious, the disease infected nine out of ten persons exposed and resulted in an estimated 3-4 million cases and an average of 495 deaths per year in the USA alone [46, 47]. According to the World Health Organization (WHO), measles remains the leading cause of vaccine-preventable deaths in children, resulting in more than 140,000 deaths in 2018 [48].

Measles is an acute viral respiratory illness caused by *Measles morbillivirus* (MeV), also called measles virus (MV). The virus (Fig. 2.10) is a single-stranded, enveloped, non-segmented RNA virus of the genus Morbillivirus within the family Paramyxoviridae [46]. Humans are the natural hosts of the virus, with no known animal reservoir.

Transmission of the measles virus occurs when a person comes in direct contact with secreted droplets from an infected person or following inhalation of air-borne viruses, spread when an infected person breathes, coughs, or sneezes. Viruses may remain infectious in room air for 2 h after an infected person leaves the area [46].

The clinical signs and symptoms of measles start 10–14 days after exposure. A prodrome of fever, malaise, cough, coryza, and conjunctivitis is generally followed by a characteristic enanthema on the mucous membranes of the mouth, which appears as bright red spots, often with a bluish-white central dot—referred to as Koplik spots (Fig. 2.11) [49].

---

[5]The recent emergence of monkeypox (now referred to as *mpox* to avoid unintended stigmata associated with the term "monkey") in the USA and elsewhere around the world highlights the potential concerns referable to the cessation of routine smallpox vaccinations. The mpox virus is a member of the *Orthopoxvirus* genus and mpox infections are preventable through smallpox vaccinations. The clinical presentation of mpox resembles that of smallpox, but generally of less severity and lower mortality [44].

Fig. 2.10 Electron micrograph of the measles virus. Photo credit: Cynthia S. Goldsmith, William Bellini. (Picture Source: https://en.wikipedia.org. CDC: Public Health Image Library)

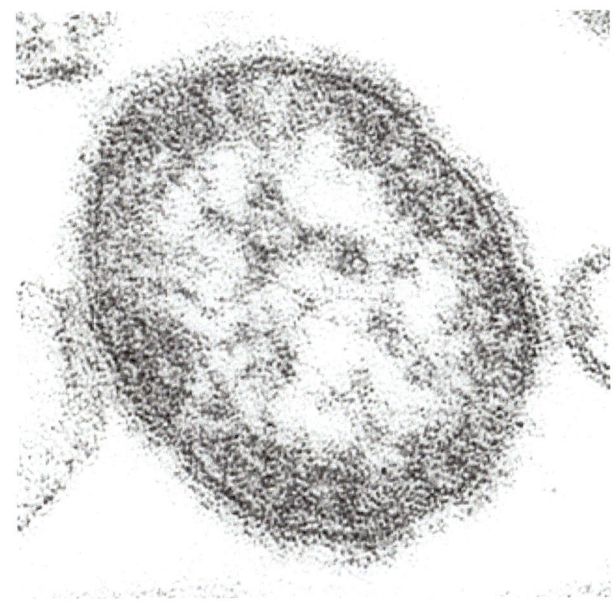

Fig. 2.11 Koplik spots. (Picture Source: https://www.cdc.gov. CDC: Public Health Image Library)

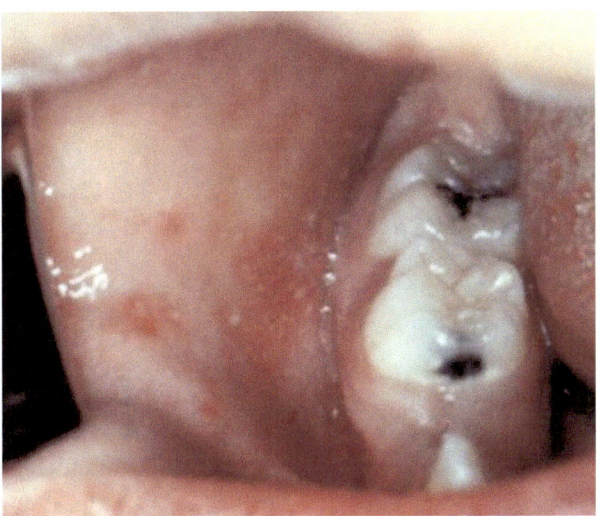

A maculopapular rash follows, which spreads from the head to the chest and back and down the legs (Fig. 2.12). A high fever (104–105 °F) often accompanies the rash [46, 49]. The rash may last around 7 days and patients are considered contagious from 4 days before to 4 days after the rash appears [46, 49].

Complications frequently associated with measles include bacterial superinfections (e.g., pneumonia, otitis media) requiring antibiotic treatment and frequently necessitating hospitalization. Serious side effects noted by the CDC also include [46, 47]:

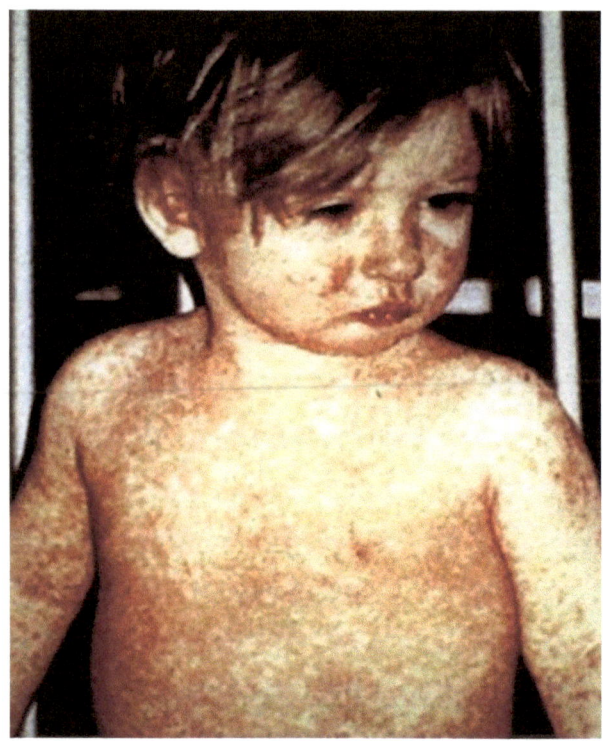

Fig. 2.12 Measles rash. (Picture Source: https://www.cdc.gov. CDC: Public Health Image Library)

- Acute encephalitis—often resulting in permanent brain damage, affecting one out of every 1000 cases.
- Death—from respiratory or neurological complications, affecting one to three of every 1000 cases
- Subacute sclerosing panencephalitis (SSPE)—a rare, but fatal degenerative disease of the central nervous system presenting 7–10 years after a measles infection.

There is no antiviral medication for measles and treatment is relegated to symptomatic supportive care. Bacterial superinfections are treated with antibiotics. Age-specific dosing with vitamin A supplementation is recommended in severe cases to help prevent eye damage and blindness, particularly among patients that may be vitamin deficient [46, 48]. Diagnosis is based on clinical presentation (Koplik spots/rash) and, in sporadic cases or new outbreaks, with laboratory confirmation using measles-specific IgM antibody tests and/or real-time polymerase chain reaction (RT-PCR) tests for measles RNA in respiratory secretions [46].

****

The mainstay of measles infection prevention is vaccination. The first measles vaccine was developed by Dr. John F. Enders (1887–1985). Following isolation of the measles virus from an 11-year-old boy (David Edmonson) at Boston Children's Hospital in 1954, Enders and his team were able to develop a live-attenuated virus vaccine. Hailed as 100%

effective following clinical trials in 1961 and licensed for public use in 1963, worldwide vaccination initiatives to stamp out measles were begun in the late 1960s [50, 51].

An improved vaccine with fewer side effects was created in 1968 by Dr. Maurice R. Hilleman (1919–2005), who in 1971 combined the vaccine with the recently developed mumps and rubella vaccines to create the ubiquitous MMR vaccine [52]. In 2005, the varicella vaccine was added to the combination, creating the MMRV vaccine, further reducing the number of injections the pediatric population had to endure in their immunization protocols, although standalone measles vaccines are still available and used in many countries [50].

A significant setback in global immunization campaigns against measles occurred in 1998 when a fraudulently researched and serially discredited paper was published in *The Lancet* asserting a link between the MMR vaccine and autism [50, 53]. Although the lead author (Andrew J. Wakefield) was subsequently censured and the article formally retracted (Fig. 2.13) by *The Lancet* [54, 55], the article added to the omnipresent undercurrent of vaccine hesitancy.

Because measles is so highly contagious, a 95% immunity among members of a community is needed to prevent an endemic outbreak [50]. *The Lancet* article fueled misinformation campaigns by anti-vaccination groups of sufficiently negative influence to trigger a drop in vaccination rates and a resurgence of cases in the UK as well as parts of the USA and Canada in the years following its publication [50].

The WHO estimates that between 2000 and 2020, 31.7 million deaths were prevented worldwide by measles vaccination [50]. However, vaccine hesitancy/complacency has resulted in increasing numbers of vulnerable persons in recent years [56–60]. WHO statistics suggest that there were 207,000 unvaccinated measles deaths globally in 2019, the highest number recorded in 23 years [50]. CDC statistics document that 1274 cases of measles were reported in the USA in 2019, the greatest number since 1992. The majority of these cases were in close-knit communities where persons were not vaccinated against measles [56].

In November 2023, the WHO/CDC issued a joint news release stating that the number of global measles cases increased by 18% and deaths by 43% in 2022 compared to 2021, mostly among children [61]. These statistics prompted John Vertefeuille, director of CDC's Global Immunization Division, to state [61]: "The increase in measles outbreaks and deaths is staggering, but, unfortunately, not unexpected given the declining vaccination rates we've seen in the past few years."

The importation of measles from overseas is of particular concern in the USA as children are increasingly forgoing vaccination and are at high risk of contracting the disease if exposed [56–60].[6] Accordingly, universal immunization is the goal of the

---

[6] In consultation with the CDC, *The Washington Post* (Lena H. Sun) reported on January 13, 2023, that more than 250,000 children who entered kindergarten in the fall of 2021 are at risk of measles because they did not receive the vaccinations required to enroll in school. A 95% vaccination coverage is required to prevent an outbreak of the highly contagious disease and, according to the CDC sources cited in the article, the current level of vaccination for measles and other vaccine-preventable diseases is the lowest in over a decade.

Early report

RETRACTED

Ileal-lymphoid-nodular hyperplasia, non-specific colitis, and pervasive developmental disorder in children

A J Wakefield, S H Murch, A Anthony, J Linnell, D M Casson, M Malik, M Berelowitz, A P Dhillon, M A Thomson, P Harvey, A Valentine, S E Davies, J A Walker-Smith

Summary

Background We investigated a consecutive series of children with chronic enterocolitis and regressive developmental disorder.

Methods 12 children (mean age 6 years [range 3–10], 11 boys) were referred to a paediatric gastroenterology unit with a history of normal development followed by loss of acquired skills, including language, together with diarrhoea and abdominal pain. Children underwent gastroenterological, neurological, and developmental assessment and review of developmental records. Ileocolonoscopy and biopsy sampling, magnetic-resonance imaging (MRI), electroencephalography (EEG), and lumbar puncture were done under sedation. Barium follow-through radiography was done where possible. Biochemical, haematological, and immunological profiles were examined.

Findings Onset of behavioural symptoms was associ[illegible] by the parents, with measles, mumps, and rub[illegible] vaccination in eight of the 12 children, with meas[illegible] infection in one child, and otitis media in a[illegible]. All 1[illegible] children had intestinal abnormalities, [illegible] from lymphoid nodular hyperplasia to a[illegible]oid u[illegible]ration. Histology showed patchy chronic infla[illegible] in 11 children and reactive ile[illegible] [illegible]erplasia in seven, but no granulomas. Be[illegible]ioural diso[illegible] included autism (nine), disintegrativ[illegible] (one), a[illegible]ossible postviral or vaccinal enc[illegible]halitis [illegible]). There were no focal neurological ab[illegible]malities and [illegible] and EEG tests were normal. Abno[illegible] laboratory results [illegible]re significantly raised urinary [illegible]thylmal[illegible] acid compared with age-matched contro[illegible], low haemoglobin in four children, [illegible] low [illegible] IgA in [illegible] children.

Interp[illegible]ation [illegible] iden[illegible] associated gastrointestinal di[illegible] and [illegible]velopmental regression in a group of previ[illegible] [illegible], which was generally associated in time [illegible] possible environmental triggers.

Lancet 199[illegible] 351: 637–41

See Commentary page

Inflammatory Bowel Disease Study Group, University Departments of Medicine and Histopathology (A J Wakefield FRCS, A Anthony MB, J Linnell PhD, A P Dhillon MRCPath, S E Davies MRCPath) **and the University Departments of Paediatric Gastroenterology** (S H Murch MB, D M Casson MRCP, M Malik MRCP, M A Thomson FRCP, J A Walker-Smith FRCP), **Child and Adolescent Psychiatry** (M Berelowitz FRCPsych), **Neurology** (P Harvey FRCP), **and Radiology** (A Valentine FRCR), **Royal Free Hospital and School of Medicine, London NW3 2QG, UK**

Correspondence to: Dr A J Wakefield

Introduction

We saw several children who, after a p[illegible] of apparent normality, lost acquired skills, inclu[illegible] com[illegible]ication. They all had gastrointestinal [illegible]mptoms, [illegible]uding abdominal pain, diarrhoea, and [illegible]ating and, i[illegible] some cases, food intolerance. We [illegible]cribe [illegible] clinical [illegible]ings, and gastrointestinal featur[illegible] of these ch[illegible]n.

Patients and met[illegible]s

12 children, co[illegible] [illegible]red to [illegible] department of paediatric gast[illegible]terology [illegible] a h[illegible]y of a pervasive developmental [illegible]der with los[illegible] [illegible]ed skills and intestinal symptoms [illegible] abdominal [illegible], bloating, and food intolerance), were inv[illegible]ated. All children were admitted to the ward f[illegible]eek, accomp[illegible]d by their parents.

[illegible]ical investigations

[illegible] took histori[illegible] including details of immunisations and [illegible] to infect[illegible] diseases, and assessed the children. In 11 ca[illegible] the histor[illegible] obtained by the senior clinician (JW-S). Neur[illegible] [illegible] psychiatric assessments were done by [illegible]sultant staff (PH, MB) with HMS-4 criteria.[1] Developmental [illegible] included a review of prospective developmental records from [illegible], health visitors, and general practitioners. Four children did not undergo psychiatric assessment in hospital; all had been assessed professionally elsewhere, so these assessments were used as the basis for their behavioural diagnosis.

After bowel preparation, ileocolonoscopy was performed by SHM or MAT under sedation with midazolam and pethidine. Paired frozen and formalin-fixed mucosal biopsy samples were taken from the terminal ileum; ascending, transverse, descending, and sigmoid colons, and from the rectum. The procedure was recorded by video or still images, and were compared with images of the previous seven consecutive paediatric colonoscopies (four normal colonoscopies and three on children with ulcerative colitis), in which the physician reported normal appearances in the terminal ileum. Barium follow-through radiography was possible in some cases.

Also under sedation, cerebral magnetic-resonance imaging (MRI), electroencephalography (EEG) including visual, brain stem auditory, and sensory evoked potentials (where compliance made these possible), and lumbar puncture were done.

Laboratory investigations

Thyroid function, serum long-chain fatty acids, and cerebrospinal-fluid lactate were measured to exclude known causes of childhood neurodegenerative disease. Urinary methylmalonic acid was measured in random urine samples from eight of the 12 children and 14 age-matched and sex-matched normal controls, by a modification of a technique described previously.[2] Chromatograms were scanned digitally on computer, to analyse the methylmalonic-acid zones from cases and controls. Urinary methylmalonic-acid concentrations in patients and controls were compared by a two-sample *t* test. Urinary creatinine was estimated by routine spectrophotometric assay.

Children were screened for antiendomyseal antibodies and boys were screened for fragile-X if this had not been done

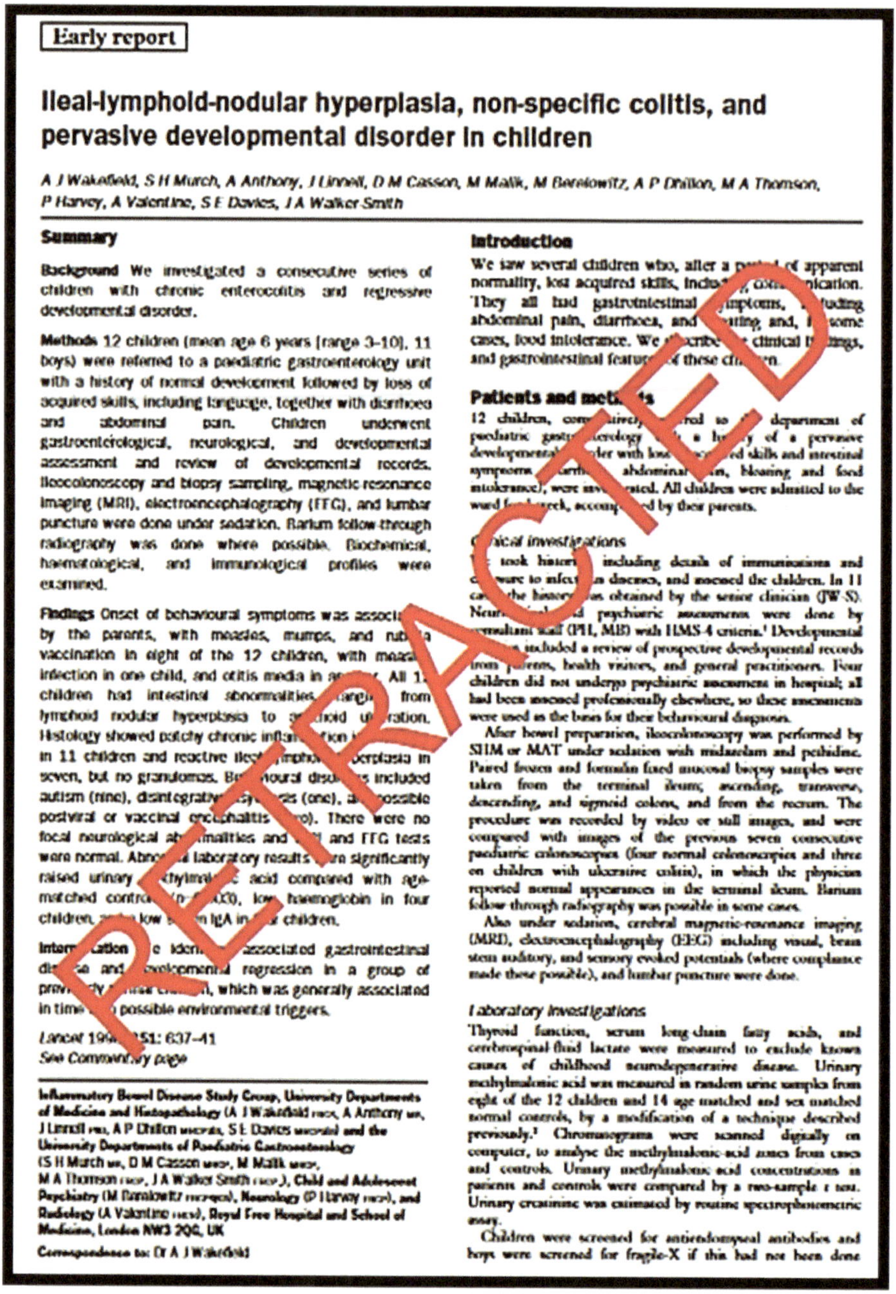

Fig. 2.13 Retracted *The Lancet* manuscript linking MMR vaccine to autism [53]. (Picture Source: https://www.sciencedirect.com)

CDC and its worldwide public health partners in the effort to end global measles outbreaks and eliminate the scourge of one of the most contagious diseases ever afflicting humankind [57].

Rubella (*German Measles, Three-day Measles*)

Like rubeola (measles), rubella was once a ubiquitous disease of childhood. Although similar in name, rubella is an entirely different disease from rubeola. Most often affecting children and young adults, rubella is a contagious viral infection caused by the RNA Rubella virus (family Togaviridae, genus *Rubivirus*). Humans are the only source of infection [62].

Most people with rubella infections have minimal or mild symptoms including a low-grade fever, sore throat, cough, swollen lymph nodes, pink eye, and headache. A rash may appear on the face and body, generally lasting around 3 days (Fig. 2.14).

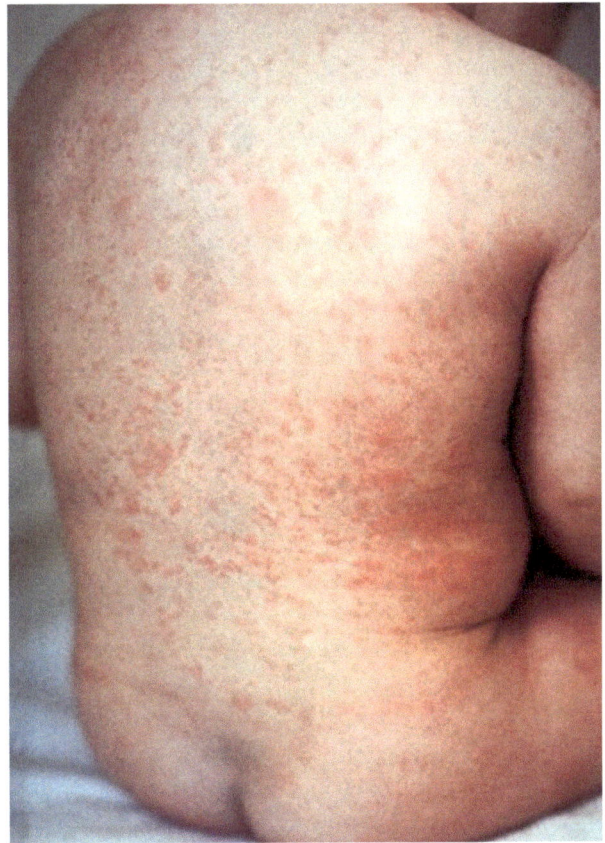

Fig. 2.14 Rubella rash on a child. (Picture Source: https://www.cdc.gov. CDC: Public Health Image Library)

Up to 70% of women who contract the disease experience arthritis-like symptoms, which are uncommon in children and men [62].

Spread of rubella occurs through virus-ladened respiratory droplets/secretions. A potentially contagious period spans the week before a rash appears and extends for around a week after the rash disappears. That said, 25–50% of patients do not develop a rash or have noticeable symptoms but are still contagious [62].

A live-attenuated rubella virus vaccine was first developed at the Merck pharmaceutical laboratories in 1969 by the prolific vaccine researcher, Dr. Maurice R. Hilleman (1919–2005). Subsequently combined with the measles and mumps vaccine, the measles-mumps-rubella (MMR) vaccine was licensed in the USA in 1971. In 1979, an improved vaccine based on the RA27/3 strain of the rubella virus, developed by Dr. Stanley A. Plotkin (1932–) at the Wistar Institute in Philadelphia, superseded the Hilleman vaccine in the MMR combination. Significant adverse side effects to the vaccine are rare, with injection site soreness, low-grade fever, rash, and muscle aches most common [63–66].

During the last major rubella outbreak in the USA in 1964–1965, there were an estimated 12.5 million cases. With the advent of the MMR vaccine—reportedly 97% effective in preventing rubella—infections are now rare in America with less than 10 people reported as having the disease per year, most having contracted the infection when traveling or living outside of the country [62, 67].

In addition to the clinical presentation, rubella infection may be confirmed by rubella IgM and IgG titers, real-time polymerase chain reaction (RT-PCR), and viral culture [62]. Treatment is relegated to supportive care.

****

The principal concern with rubella is when the disease occurs in a pregnant woman, potentially resulting in a miscarriage or fetal death. If infected early in the pregnancy, a woman has a 90% chance of passing the virus to the fetus [66]. Developing fetuses are highly susceptible to the rubella virus and are at risk of severe birth defects—referred to as congenital rubella syndrome (CRS). According to the CDC [68] and NIH [67], common birth defects from CRS include:

- Congenital heart defects
- Deafness
- Cataracts
- Microcephaly
- Intellectual disabilities (including autism)
- Liver and spleen damage
- Low birth weight
- Diabetes and thyroid disease

Children with CRS should be considered contagious for a year after birth (unless definitively demonstrated otherwise) and isolated accordingly [67]. As the rubella vaccine contains a live virus, pregnant women should not be vaccinated, according to the CDC [68], and those of child-bearing age should avoid pregnancy until 4 weeks after receiving an MMR vaccine. As there is no treatment for CRS, termination of an exposed pregnancy in an unvaccinated woman might be considered, based on local abortion legislation and parental choice [67].

CDC data indicates that during the 1964–1965 rubella epidemic in the USA, 11,000 pregnant women lost their babies, 2100 newborns died, and 20,000 babies were born with CRS [62]. As rubella is the leading cause of vaccine-preventable birth defects [66], it is imperatively self-evident that the preventive vaccine initiative which began in the USA in 1969 continues unabated.

Tuberculosis (*Phthisis, White Death, Consumption, Scrofula*)

On March 24, 1882, Dr. Robert Koch correctly announced that he had identified the tubercle bacillus responsible for tuberculosis (TB), known today as *Mycobacterium tuberculosis* [69, 70]. A disease as ancient as mankind, tuberculosis killed one out of every seven people living in the USA and Europe in the 1800s [71] and over time may have killed more persons than any other microbial pathogen [72].

Referred to by a variety of names and epithets over the ages [71, 72], including the "Captain of All These Men of Death," the tuberculosis bacillus usually attacks the lungs but may also infect extra-pulmonary body parts, such as the kidney, spine (Pott disease), and brain. As not everyone with a tuberculosis infection gets sick, two classes of infection are currently recognized: latent TB infection (LTBI) and (active) TB disease [73]. Additionally, as the bacillus' antibiotic resistance has increased over recent years, infections are now labeled as drug-susceptible, drug-resistant, multidrug-resistant, and extensively drug-resistant [71].

An uncommon form of the disease, referred to as "scrofula" during the Middle Ages, infects the lymph nodes in the neck (Fig. 2.15), generally as a secondary dissemination of pulmonary TB or, rarely, following a primary infection of the adenoids or tonsils [71, 74].

The tuberculosis bacillus is spread by air-borne droplets from an infected person with pulmonary disease following a cough, sneeze, or talking/shouting. Aerosolized bacteria inhaled into the lungs of a non-infected person can seed a pulmonary infection and/or disseminate through the bloodstream to other parts of the body, causing infections in the kidney, brain, or spine. Pulmonary infections are contagious; infections in other parts of the body are generally not [73].

The symptoms of TB disease depend on the disease location. Active pulmonary tuberculosis is the most common type and is characterized by cough, chest pain, and hemoptysis (blood in the cough exudate). Fever, chills, weight loss, night sweats, and fatigue are common accompanying symptoms. A chest X-ray typically shows a suggestive parenchymal infiltrate, cavitary pulmonary lesion, hilar adenopathy or pleural effusion, often in combination. Skin and blood tests are almost always positive for infection, and sputum smears and/or cultures are generally definitive for the infecting bacterium [73, 75].

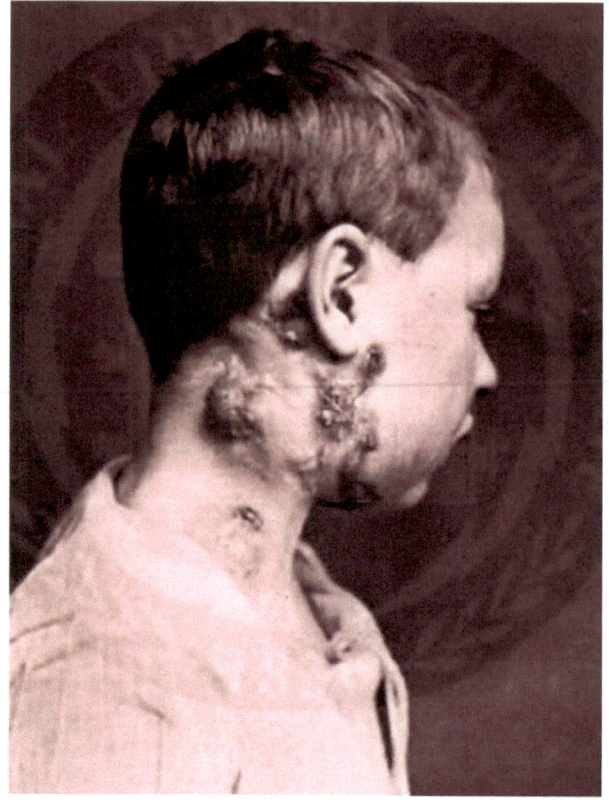

Fig. 2.15 Scrofula of the neck. From: Bramwell, Byrom Edinburgh, Constable, 1893 Atlas of Clinical Medicine. (Picture Source: https://en. wikipedia.org. National Library of Medicine, NIH)

In contrast, patients with latent TB infections are not sick and have no symptoms. In the latent state, live bacteria are sequestered in the lung(s) by the patient's immune/inflammatory response and may remain harbored in an inactive state for a lifetime without causing disease. Generally, the latent patient will have a positive skin or blood test but is not contagious to others. Fibrotic scars or (calcified) nodules/granulomas may be evident on a chest X-ray. In some cases, particularly if the immune system is compromised by an ancillary illness (e.g., diabetes, substance abuse, HIV), the sequestered/inactive bacteria may become active, multiply, and cause TB disease [73, 75].

Both skin and blood tests are available to detect latent and active TB. The Mantoux tuberculin skin test (TST) is the front-line method of determining whether a person is infected with *M. tuberculosis*. The TST is performed by an intradermal injection of 0.1 ml of tuberculin purified protein derivative (PPD), developed by Florence Seibert (1897–1991) in the 1930s [76]. The size of the ensuing inflammatory reaction is measured 48 hours later and is considered positive if the diameter of induration is 15 mm or more in a patient with no known risk factors for TB. Lesser diameters of induration are considered positive in patients with a high risk of exposure or are immunocompromised [77].

Interferon-gamma release assays (IGRAs) are whole-blood tests that can aid in diagnosing TB infection by measuring a person's immune reactivity to *M.*

tuberculosis antigens. Like skin tests, they do not differentiate latent tuberculosis infection from tuberculosis disease. Two such tests are currently licensed for use in the USA. A negative chest X-ray in the presence of positive skin or blood test suggests extra-pulmonary tuberculosis [73, 77].

With respect to pulmonary tuberculosis, the presence of acid-fast bacilli (AFB) on a sputum smear suggests tuberculosis but does not clinch the diagnosis as some acid-fast bacilli are not *M. tuberculosis*. However, a positive culture for *M. tuberculosis* affords a definitive diagnosis [73, 77].

With the introduction of streptomycin in 1943 [78], antibiotic administration became the mainstay of treatment for TB. However, over ensuing years drug-resistant strains emerged, necessitating alternative drug regimens. Currently, rifampin, isoniazid, pyrazinamide, and ethambutol are commonly used in sequential dosing regimens or in combination protocols over several months, with the possible substitution of other drugs depending on the antibiotic resistance of the infecting organism. Both latent and active infections are appropriately treated with antibiotics. In the presence of multiple-resistant organisms and/or the existence of ancillary illnesses (diabetes, HIV/AIDS), treatment regimens may be prolonged, involve multiple drugs, and generally fall in the province of a tuberculosis infectious disease expert [71, 73, 78].

In 1921, the Bacillus Calmette-Guérin (BCG) vaccine, developed by Albert Calmette (1863–1933) and Jean-Marie Camille Guerin (1872–1961), became available for human administration. BCG is a live-attenuated form of *Mycobacterium bovis* which is helpful in preventing some forms of tuberculosis. Not widely used in the USA, the vaccine is administered to infants and small children in developing countries where TB is endemic. Its principal efficacy is in the prevention of TB meningitis and disseminated (miliary) tuberculosis. It does not prevent primary infection and does not prevent reactivation of latent pulmonary infections. Additionally, it plays an ancillary role in the treatment of bladder cancer and is used as a vaccine against leprosy, with established clinical efficacy in both instances. Persons who have received the BCG vaccine will routinely show a positive skin test for TB, necessitating the use of blood tests for screening purposes [71, 79–81].

****

An interesting facet of tuberculosis treatment in the pre-antibiotic era was the introduction of the TB sanitarium. Based on the "curative" principles of fresh (cold/mountain) air, bed rest, and nutritious food, sanitariums for the treatment of TB flourished in the mid-nineteenth to the mid-twentieth centuries in the USA and abroad [82].

In America, the first TB sanitarium was established in 1875 by Joseph Gleitsmann (1840–1914) in Ashville, NC, followed by Dr. Edward L. Trudeau's (1848–1915) famous Adirondack Cottage Sanatorium in Saranac Lake, NY, in 1884 (Fig. 2.16). By 1904 there were 115 sanitariums in the USA and by 1953 there were 839 sanitariums with a capacity for 136,000 patients [71].

During the sanitarium era, multiple ancillary experimental surgical interventions were used to treat pulmonary tuberculosis. Among them were artificial

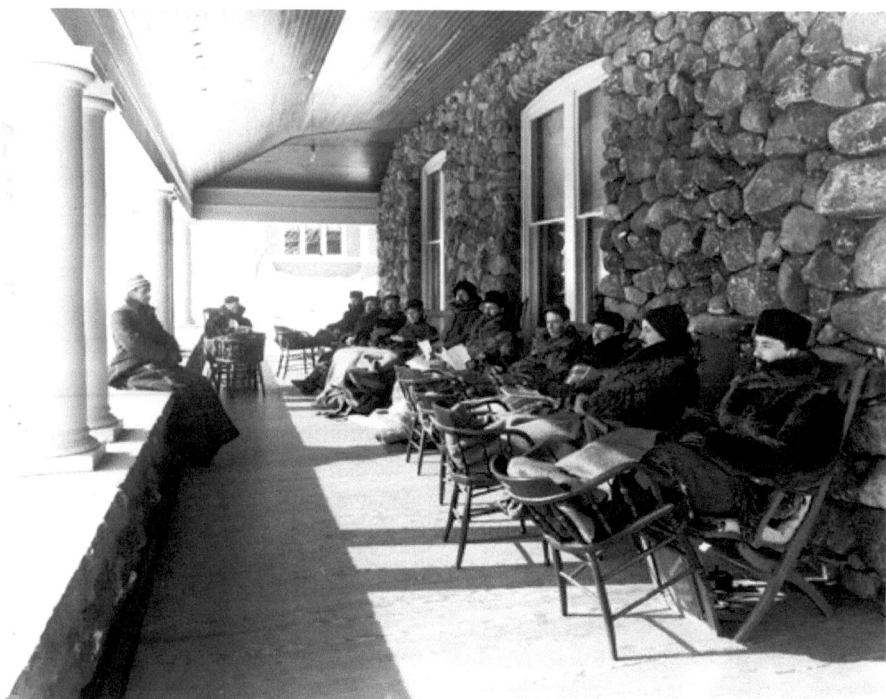

Fig. 2.16 Trudeau's "fresh air" sanatorium. Circa 1886. (Picture Source: https://adhstudiotds. wordpress.com. Saranac Lake Free Library)

pneumothoraces, thoracoplasty, plombage, phrenic nerve crush, and partial lung resections. Hundreds of thousands of these procedures were performed over the years, but none was rigorously tested in randomized clinical trials [83, 84].

To raise money for TB sanitariums, the American social worker Emily P. Bissel (1861–1948) started the "Christmas Seals" initiative in 1907 (Fig. 2.17)—a program which is still active and supported by the American Lung Association [85].

From today's perspective, it seems unlikely that sanitarium treatment provided any true curative benefit, although some patients may have converted to an inactive/ latent state. Be that as it may, the movement was probably of some societal value in that it quarantined contagious individuals.

In 1956, clinical researcher Dr. Wallace Fox (1920–2010) moved to India as the director of the Tuberculosis Chemotherapy Center in Madras to explore the need for hospital/sanitarium isolation when antibiotic drugs—isoniazid and para-amino salicylic (PAS)—were administered. The trial showed no advantage for a sanitarium group, and no added risk of infection for family contacts of those treated at home [86, 87]. The study brought a precipitous end to the sanitarium movement around the world, which was largely untenable from the beginning in that the number of patients in need of tuberculosis treatment far outnumbered the availability and affordability of sanitarium beds, particularly in third-world countries [82].

Fig. 2.17 Poster commissioned by the American Lung Association to promote sales of Christmas Seals. Circa 1926. Artist: George V. Curtis. (Picture Source: https://www.atsjournals. org. American Lung Association)

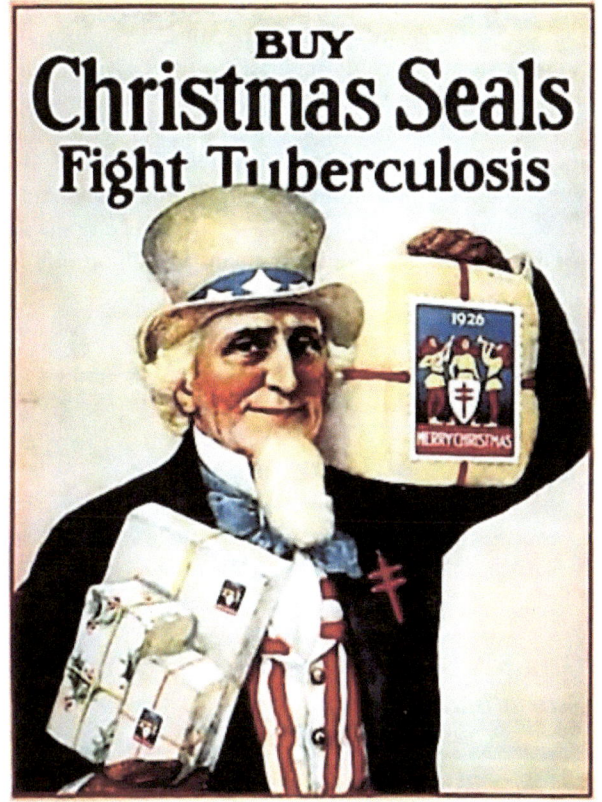

Unlike sanitarium treatment, surgery retains a limited adjunctive role in multidrug-resistant pulmonary disease and in some cases of spinal tuberculosis, abscess formation, and tuberculous destruction of weight bearing joints, among other related conditions [83, 84, 88].

****

Although the worldwide incidence of tuberculosis has declined in recent decades [89], a substantial uptick in cases occurred during the COVID-19 epidemic, according to recently published WHO estimates [90]. Moreover, CDC and WHO data document ongoing concerns referable to persistent/undiagnosed cases in the USA and abroad and the ever-increasing presence of multidrug-resistant TB [91, 92].

According to the WHO, an estimated 10.6 million people fell ill with tuberculosis in 2022 and a total of 1.3 million people died [92]. Alarmingly, the WHO also estimates that only two in five people with drug-resistant TB accessed medical treatment in 2022 [92]—potentially harboring an enormous reservoir of resistant bacteria among the untreated. People living with HIV are uniquely susceptible to TB infection and the combination is often lethal. According to the WHO, around 167,000 people died of HIV-associated TB in 2022 [92].

In 1953, there were 84,304 reported cases of TB in the USA with an incidence rate of 52.6 cases per 100,000 persons, according to CDC data [73]. By 2021, the number of active cases reported to the CDC had dropped to 7882 (2.4 cases per 100,000), with an estimated 13 million people living with latent TB [73].

The WHO notes that 98% of currently reported cases are in low- and middle-income countries and that current spending is less than half of that needed for worldwide TB prevention, diagnosis, and treatment. Ending the TB epidemic by 2030 is one of the initiatives of the United Nations Sustainable Development Goals (SDGs) but requires adequate financial support, not currently available [92, 93].

N.B.
The reader might enjoy reading the experiential anecdotes of persons suffering from tuberculosis found in Sheila M. Rothman's book: *Living in the Shadow of Death: Tuberculosis and the Social Experience of Illness in American History* (Johns Hopkins University Press, Baltimore, MD, 1995) and/or Shirley Morgan's book: *Well Diary … I Have Tuberculosis: Researching a Teenager's 1918 Sanatorium Experience* (author published).

Group A Streptococcal Disease (*Scarlet Fever, Scarlatina, Quincy*)

Hardly a Victorian-era novel or motion picture is written without a chapter or scene depicting a sick child suffering from scarlet fever.[7] Once an enormously prevalent and serious disease, scarlet fever is caused by a group A hemolytic streptococcus bacterium, specifically *Streptococcus pyogenes* (Fig. 2.18) [94, 95].

The streptococcus bacteria causing scarlet fever is the same as that causing the ubiquitous "strep throat" infection of childhood. The distinction is that the strain of bacteria causing scarlet fever secretes an erythrogenic ("redness-producing") toxin, referred to as scarlet fever toxin or "Dick toxin," after American physician and pathologist Georg F. Dick and his wife, Gladys H. Dick, who identified the hemolytic streptococcus and associated toxin causing scarlet fever in 1923 [94].

In addition to the fever, chills, sore throat, swollen glands, whitish pharyngeal exudate, and body aches of strep throat, the hallmark of scarlet fever is a characteristic rash with fine bumps that feel like sandpaper (Fig. 2.19). The rash commonly appears 1–2 days after the illness begins and spreads from the neck region all over the body and begins to fade at around 7 days, often leaving peeling skin behind [94–96].

---

[7] For example: *Little Women*, by Louisa May Alcott, depicts Beth March's death by scarlet fever in both book (1868/69) and movie versions (2019).

Fig. 2.18 "Chain-like" *Streptococcus pyogenes* bacteria (900× mag). (Picture Source: https://en.wikipedia.org. CDC: Public Health Image Library)

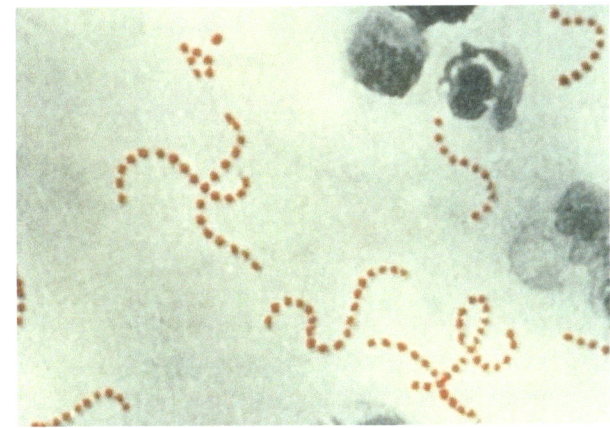

Fig. 2.19 Scarlet fever rash. (Picture Source: https://en.wikipedia.org. Wikimedia Commons: Badobadop)

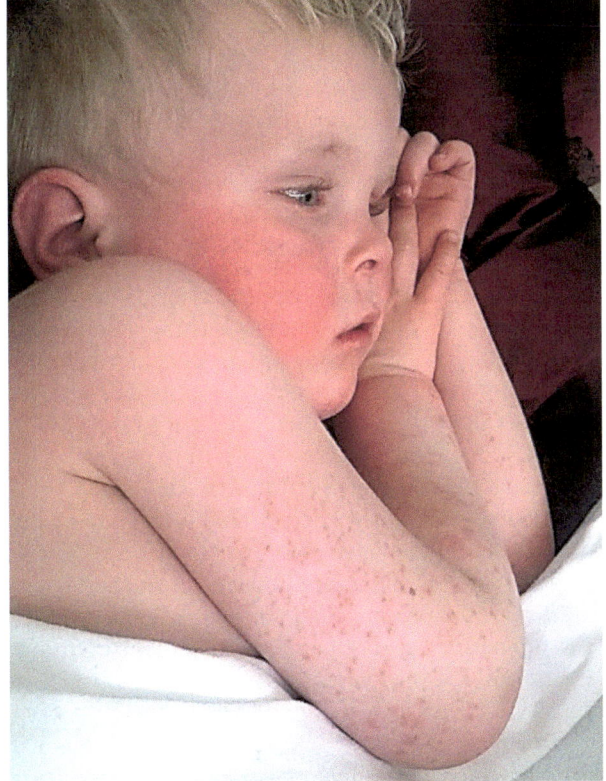

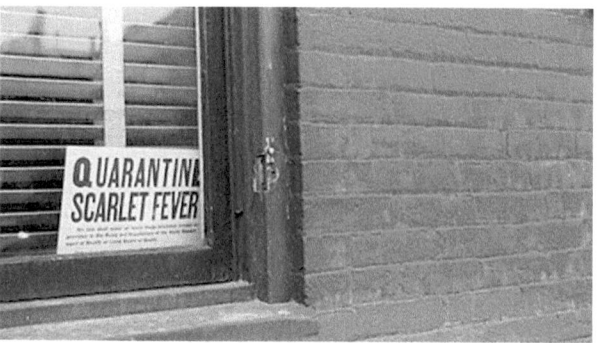

Fig. 2.20 Scarlet fever quarantine sign, Circa 1940. (Picture Source: https://asm.org. Wikimedia Commons)

The streptococcal bacteria which cause scarlet fever are most commonly spread through respiratory droplets (talking, coughing, sneezing) and are highly contagious. In the pre-antibiotic era, scarlet fever was a frequent cause of debilitating illness and death, generally in preadolescent children ages 5–15 years. To prevent outbreaks of disease, infected persons were routinely quarantined (Fig. 2.20) [94, 95].

Following the ready availability of penicillin in the mid-1940s, providing a rapid and effective treatment for strep infections, scarlet fever faded from the public consciousness. However, recent outbreaks in Europe and the USA, without clear explanation, are a cause of current concern [94].

****

One of the sequelae of an untreated or inadequately treated group A strep infections is rheumatic fever, providing the imperative for a complete course of curative antibiotics. Rheumatic fever is not an infection but an inflammatory reaction to the antecedent step infection bacteria. Antibodies generated to fight the streptococcus organism inappropriately attack healthy tissue as well, including heart muscle and valves, joints, skin, and nerves [97, 98].

Symptoms of rheumatic fever include fever, fatigue, joint pain, chest pain, heart palpitations, and jerky, uncontrolled body movements (Sydenham chorea), among others. The inflammatory reactions to skin and joints are generally short lived but may last for several months in the heart and nervous system (chorea) [97, 98].

Heart inflammation can permanently damage the heart valves causing a characteristic murmur, regurgitation, or stenosis—referred to as rheumatic heart disease. Heart failure or arrhythmias may ensue and if sufficiently severe may necessitate surgery or result in death [97, 98].

Treatment of rheumatic fever is centered on eliminating the infecting streptococcal bacteria with antibiotics (penicillin/amoxicillin). High doses of concomitant anti-inflammatory medications are almost always indicated as well, usually with aspirin (or other nonsteroidal anti-inflammatory drugs) in conjunction with steroids if heart inflammation is severe. Prolonged prophylactic antibiotic administration may also be indicated to guard against recurrent strep infections [97, 98].

Varicella (*Chickenpox*)

Chickenpox (or varicella) is a highly contagious disease caused by the varicella-zoster virus (VZV), infecting up to 90% of persons who are not immune and come in close contact with an infected individual. Before the varicella vaccine was introduced in 1995, approximately 4 million people contracted chickenpox each year in the USA, 10,500 were hospitalized, and 100–150 people died, according to the CDC [99]. With the current vaccination recommendations, cases of chickenpox have dropped 97% and hospitalization and deaths have become rare [99].

Transmission of the varicella virus, which infects only humans, occurs via aerosolized droplets from an infected individual or by direct contact with the pustular skin lesions characteristic of the disease [100]. In adults, a viral prodrome of fever, lethargy, and body aches generally proceeds onset of the prototypical itchy rash with fluid-filled blisters (Fig. 2.21). In children, the rash may be the presenting sign of the disease.

The varicella rash generally starts on the scalp or face and then spreads to the trunk and extremities and may involve the mouth, eyelids, and genital area. Typically, the rash blisters scab over at about 1 week and begin to heal and disappear at around the 2-week mark [99, 101].

Fig. 2.21 Varicella rash. (Picture Source: https://www.cdc.gov. CDC: Public Health Image Library)

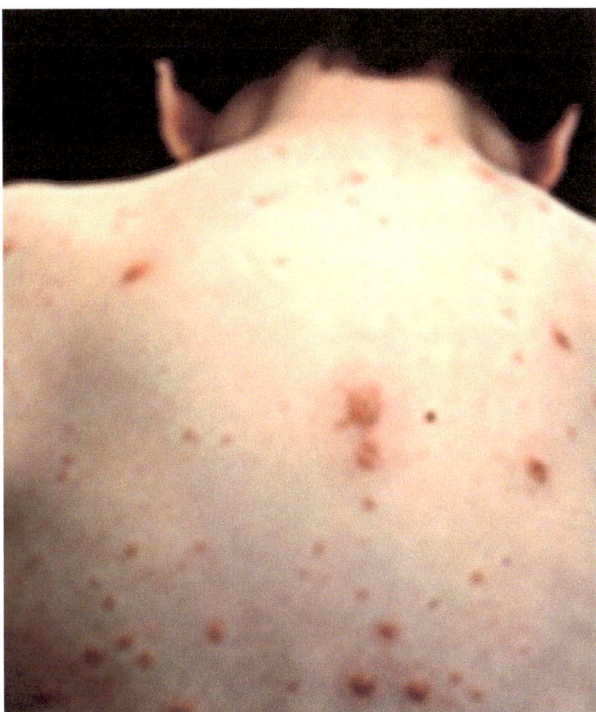

Although serious complications from chickenpox are relatively rare in healthy people, those at higher risk include: infants, adolescents, adults, pregnant women, and persons who are immunocompromised (HIV/AIDS, cancer, transplants, chemotherapy, etc.). Complications include skin infections (most common in children), pneumonia (Fig. 2.22) (most common in adults), encephalitis, hemorrhage, sepsis, and death in some instances [99].

Be that as it may, in the years before a vaccine was available (1995), parents frequently held "chickenpox parties" to purposefully expose their preschoolers to the disease through play with an infected child. The rationale was that the disease was ubiquitous and inevitable and best dealt with at an age where serious complications were relatively rare and would not disrupt school-time if acquired later.

Although the practice is still embraced by some anti-vaxxers as a natural means to build long-lasting immunity in their children [102], the concept is outdated and irresponsible at this time and forcefully discouraged by the CDC and other health agencies [99]. The reason is simple. A vaccine is available which is safe and effective and has minimal side effects. A native infection is a gamble with serious and unpredictable complications and, at minimum, subjects a child to a debilitating illness, even if relatively short-lived.

Based on pervasive disease and societal burden, the USA was the first country to implement a routine varicella vaccination program following licensure of the live, attenuated varicella vaccine (VARIVAX, Merck & Co, Inc) in 1995 [99, 103]. The vaccine is currently administered in a two-dose regime during early childhood and is 70–90% effective in preventing varicella and 95% effective in preventing severe varicella, with breakthrough infections generally having a very mild symptom

Fig. 2.22 Varicella
pneumonia. (Picture
Source: https://www.cdc.
gov/chickenpox. CDC)

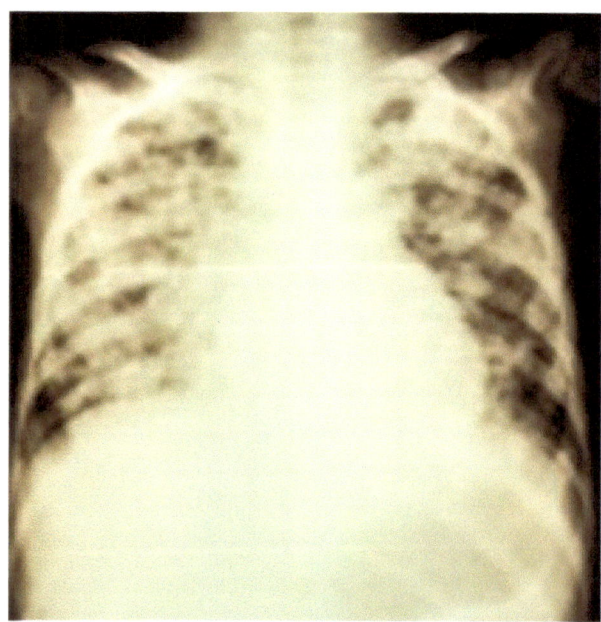

complex [99, 104]. To simplify childhood immunization scheduling, the vaccine is typically given in conjunction with the MMR vaccine, forming the current MMRV (measles, mumps, rubella, and varicella) vaccine combination [105].

Treatment of varicella infections is symptomatic with topical lotions used to relieve pruritus (itching) and acetaminophen to reduce fever. In patients at risk for severe complications, antiviral medications (acyclovir or valacyclovir) may be indicated [99]. Of particular note is the avoidance of aspirin in children, as there is an associated risk of developing Reye's syndrome [106] when aspirin is taken in conjunction with influenza, chickenpox, and other viral infections.

****

After a person recovers from chickenpox, the varicella zoster virus (VZV) remains dormant (inactive) within the dorsal root ganglia of peripheral or cranial nerve cells, often for years or decades. When reactivated (by a poorly understood mechanism), the virus travels along the nerve bodies to the skin, producing a painful rash, known as herpes zoster or *shingles* [107, 108].

Generally, the shingles rash develops as a stripe on one side of the body or face (Fig. 2.23) with blisters that scab over in 7–10 days and clears up in 2–4 weeks. A prodrome of pain, itching, or tingling may occur before the rash appears. In persons with a weakened immune system, the rash may be more widespread. If involving

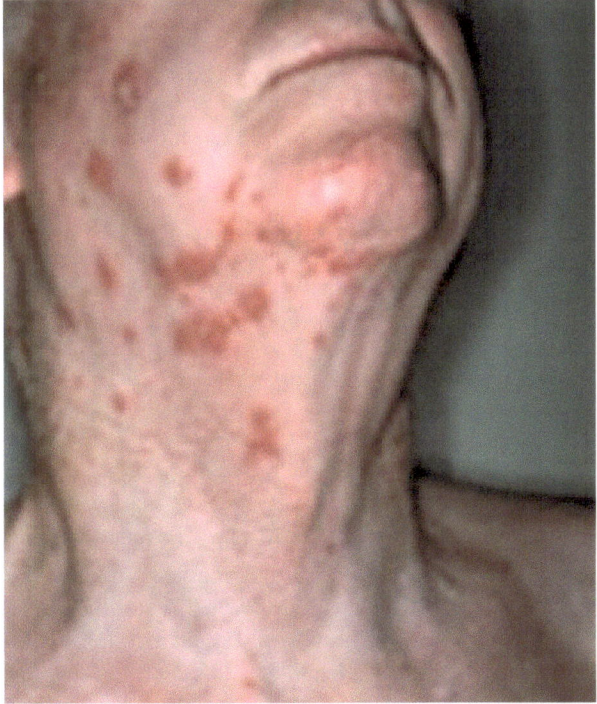

Fig. 2.23 Shingles rash involving the face. (Picture Source: https://www.cdc. gov. CDC: Public Health Image Library)

the face, there is risk for eye damage and blindness. Similarly, hearing loss may occur if there is involvement around the ears [107, 108].

The most common complication of shingles is postherpetic neuralgia (PHN), which is characterized by severe pain in the area of the shingles rash. PHN pain usually resolves within weeks or months but may last for years, creating a significant impediment to daily living in those so affected [108].

Shingles, itself, is not contagious but chickenpox can be transmitted to a non-immune individual if contact is made with the exudate from the shingles rash. Anyone who has had chickenpox is at risk of shingles, but the incidence is greatest in persons over 50 years of age. Approximately 1 million cases of shingles are diagnosed each year in the USA, occurring in about 10% of persons with a prior history of chickenpox. Although rare, it is possible to get shingles more than once [108, 109].

Like chickenpox, treatment of shingles is symptomatic. Antiviral medications may make the duration of an attack shorter and less severe and may lessen the chance of PHN if taken early in the course of the disease [108].

Similarly, the mainstay of shingles prevention is vaccination. The CDC recommends that adults 50 years of age or older with a prior history of chickenpox get vaccinated with two doses of the recombinant zoster vaccine called *Shingrix*. (As of 2020, the *Zostavax* vaccine is no longer available for use in the USA.) The Shingrix vaccine is more than 90% effective in preventing shingles and PHN in persons with a healthy immune system and remains protective for at least 7 years after immunization. Persons vaccinated for chickenpox are at low risk of developing shingles [109, 110].

Diphtheria (*Boulogne Sore Throat, "The Strangler of Children," Throat Distemper*)

Known as "the strangler of children," diphtheria was a relentless epidemic killer—principally of children—in the USA and throughout the world (Fig. 2.24) until an effective cure and vaccine became available and widely used in the 1920s [111].

The *Corynebacterium diphtheriae* bacillus was first identified as the causative bacteria of diphtheria by Edwin Klebs (1834–1913) and Friedrich August Johannes Löffler (1852–1915) in 1883/84 [111, 112]. Principally infecting the respiratory tract, with a resultant fever, sore throat, and swollen glands in the neck, some strains of the bacterium secrete a noxious toxin which was subsequently identified as the causative agent responsible for the high mortality rate associated with diphtheria infections [113].

The *C. diphtheriae* toxin can attack and damage multiple organ systems (heart, kidney, nerves), but the pathognomonic reaction is the formation of a gray pseudomembrane in the oropharynx, which of sufficient size may obstruct respiration (most commonly in children) and result in a slow agonizing asphyxiation (Fig. 2.25). Historically, around one in ten infected children died from the disease, with a

Fig. 2.24 A ghostly skeleton, representing diphtheria, trying to strangle a sick child. Artist: Richard Tennant Cooper, 1885–1957. (Picture Source: https://artsci.case.edu/dittrick. Wellcome Collection)

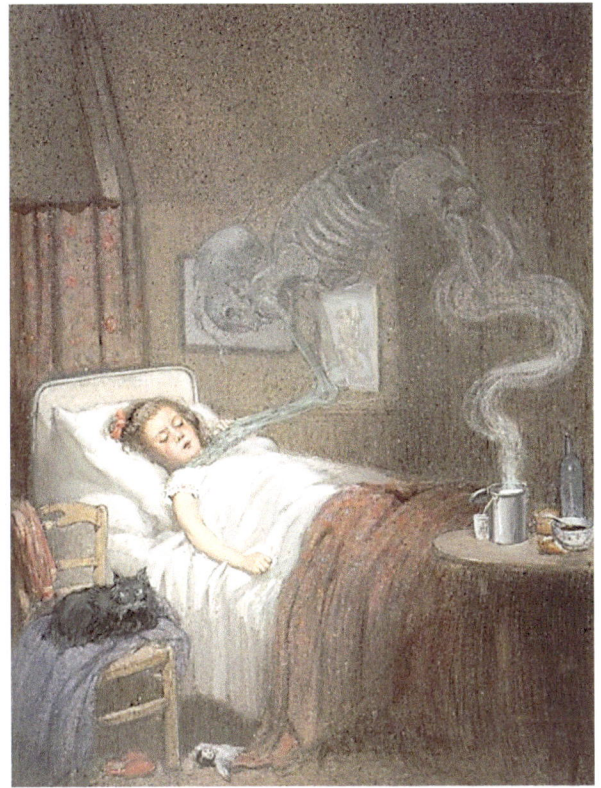

staggering case-fatality ratio of almost 40% in a 1735 epidemic which swept through New England. Regarded as a likely death sentence, 206,000 cases of diphtheria were recorded in the USA in 1921, resulting in 15,520 deaths [111].

In addition to diphtheria respiratory infections, most commonly spread person-to-person through pulmonary droplets (cough, sneeze), there is a cutaneous form of the disease, resulting in a slowly healing rash or ulcer (Fig. 2.26). Highly contagious through direct contact or environmental bacterial contamination, systemic complications are comparatively rare and spontaneous resolution generally takes place over several weeks or months [114, 115].

****

One of the earliest forms of treatment for diphtheria was a tracheotomy, which involves surgically cutting a hole in the trachea and inserting a tube through the hole to allow unobstructed passage of air to the lungs and to facilitate the removal of secretions [111, 116]. In 1890, Shibasaburo Kitasato (1852–1931) and Emil von Behring (1854–1917) developed a diphtheria antitoxin, derived from serum that was drawn from horses which had been inoculated with the diphtheria toxin (Fig. 2.27).

Fig. 2.25 Illustration of the diphtheria pseudomembrane. From: *A Practical Guide to Health/* Review and Harold Publisher, 1910. (Picture Source: https://www. smithsonianmag.com)

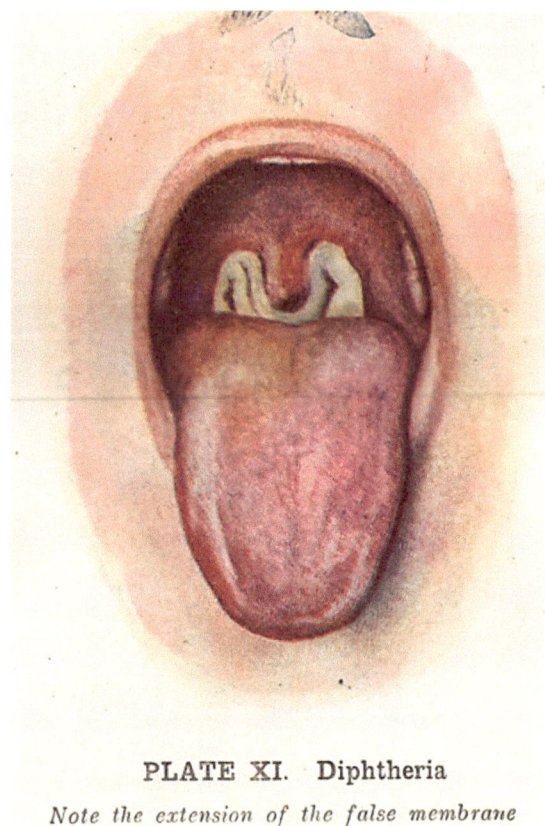

PLATE XI. Diphtheria

*Note the extension of the false membrane
to the soft palate*

Fig. 2.26 A diphtheria skin lesion on the leg. (Picture Source: https:// phil.cdc.gov. CDC: Public Health Image Library)

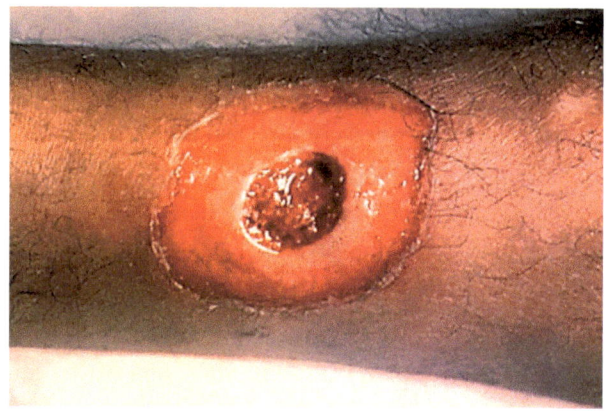

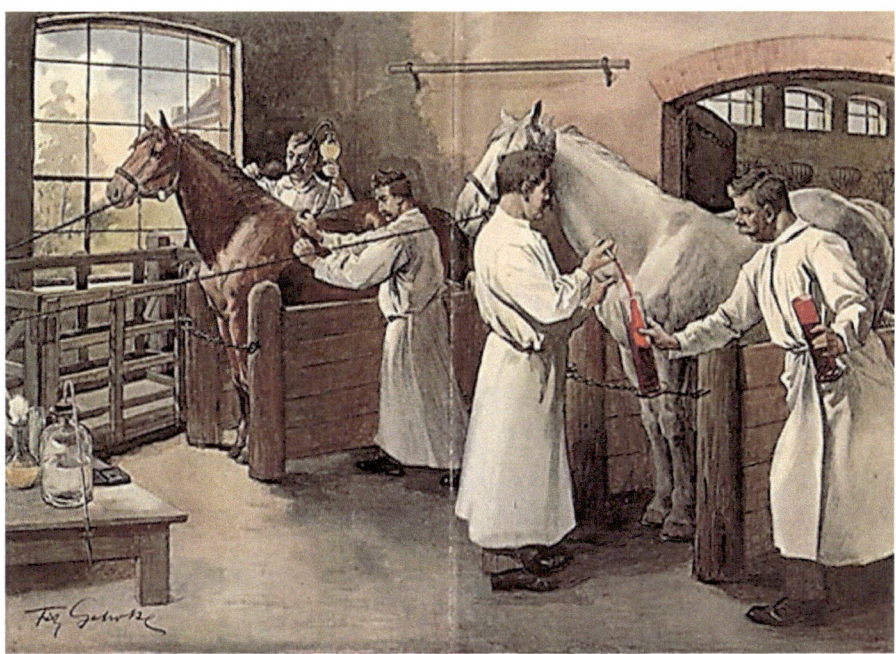

Fig. 2.27 Painting of horses being bled for serum, circa 1900. Artist: Fritz Gehrke. (Picture Source: https://www.nlm.nih.gov. National Library of Medicine)

Antibodies produced by the inoculated horses neutralized the diphtheria toxin, mitigating its toxic effects [115, 116].

Without question, antitoxin horse serum saved lives but had drawbacks of its own. First, producing enough horse serum for global distribution was a non-sequitur and ready availability was always problematic. Second, maintaining sterility was difficult and instances of disease transmission via contaminated serum were well documented. Third, people frequently developed an immune response to the horse serum itself, experiencing rash, swelling, fever, and joint pains, subsequently referred to as *serum sickness*[8] [111].

Vaccines for diphtheria soon followed the introduction of horse serum antitoxin. Initially, combinations of toxin and antitoxin were used, but in 1924 Gaston Ramon (1886–1963) developed a diphtheria toxoid, consisting of neutralized (inactivated) diphtheria toxin, that proved to impart permanent diphtheria immunity with minimal side effects. Currently produced from toxigenic *C. diphtheriae* grown in liquid media, toxoid diphtheria vaccines are still in use today and are generally given in combination with other vaccines, such as tetanus toxoid and pertussis (DTaP) [111, 117].

---

[8] Of note, a horse serum antitoxin is still available through the CDC under an Investigational New Drug Protocol (IND) and is indicated for use in active cases of pulmonary tuberculosis [117].

Of scientific interest, it is now known that the toxin producing strains of the *C. diphtheriae* bacillus are, themselves, infected (lysogenized) with a viral bacterio-phage that transfers the genetic information (*tox* gene) to the bacterium for the pro-duction of the characteristic toxin [115].

****

The diagnosis of diphtheria is based on clinical presentation coupled with culture isolation of the *C. diphtheriae* bacillus from the nares or oropharynx or from cutane-ous lesions, as indicated. Confirmatory tests such as polymerase chain reaction (PCR) are also available. Positive identification of toxin producing strains is done with an immunoprecipitation test, known as the Elek test [118], performed exclu-sively in the USA by the CDC's Pertussis and Diphtheria Laboratory at this time [115].

Lifesaving treatment of respiratory diphtheria is imperatively initiated based on a presumptive clinical diagnosis, with administration of antitoxin and antibiotics (erythromycin or penicillin) without waiting for culture results or other confirmatory tests. Respiratory support is utilized, as needed. Antibiotics alone are usually ade-quate for cutaneous cases. As diphtheria infection may not confer lifelong immunity, vaccination with diphtheria toxoid is recommended during convalescence [115].

With the vaccination initiative started in the 1920s, diphtheria cases have virtu-ally disappeared in the USA [111, 119]. At this time, diphtheria occurs only spo-radically or in small outbreaks throughout the world in areas where the disease remains endemic, according to the PAHO/WHO [120]. That said, like so many other diseases in the current era of vaccine skepticism and hesitancy, cases have started to re-emerge [121].

Pertussis (*Whooping Cough*)

Pertussis is an extremely contagious pulmonary disease caused by the *Bordetella pertussis* bacterium. The bacterium produces toxins that paralyze the cilia of the respiratory epithelial cells, inhibiting the clearing of secretions and inflaming the respiratory tract. Over several weeks, the characteristic cough becomes progres-sively more severe with resultant paroxysms of severe coughing (Fig. 2.28), often followed by a constricted inspiratory effort producing the characteristic high-pitched "whoop" [122–124].

Spread of the *B. pertussis* bacterium from person-to-person occurs through respiratory droplets expelled during a cough or sneeze. Following the usual incuba-tion period of 7–10 days, the clinical course is generally divided into three stages (Fig. 2.29) [122, 123]:

- The initial or catarrhal stage is characterized by cold-like symptoms with low-grade fever, runny nose, sneezing, and a mild cough.
- After 1–2 weeks, the cough becomes more severe with rapid bursts of coughing, referred to as the paroxysmal stage. Frequently lasting 2–3 or more weeks,

Fig. 2.28 Young boy with
a pertussis cough/whoop.
(Picture Source: http://phil.
cdc.gov. CDC: Public
Health Image Library)

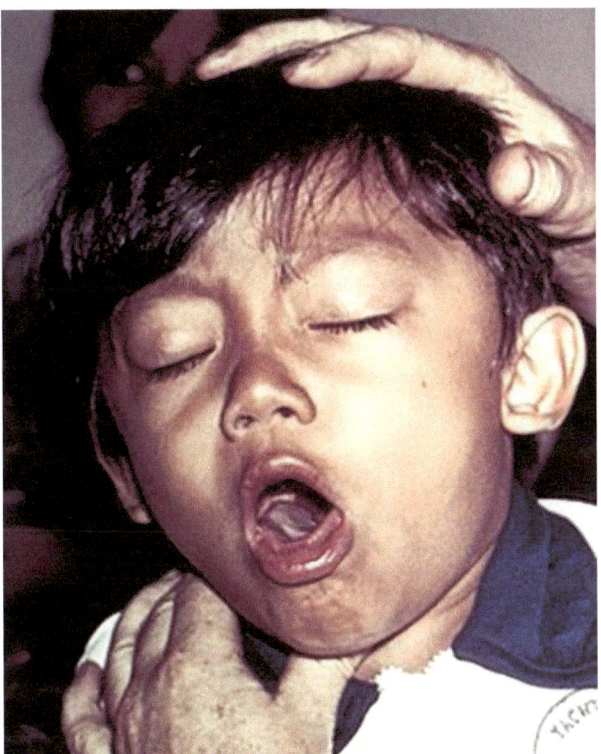

Whooping Cough Disease Progression

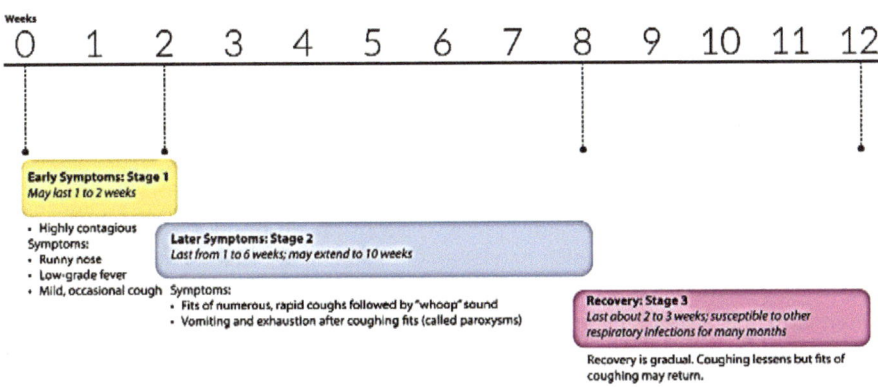

Early Symptoms: Stage 1
May last 1 to 2 weeks

- Highly contagious
Symptoms:
- Runny nose
- Low-grade fever
- Mild, occasional cough

Later Symptoms: Stage 2
Last from 1 to 6 weeks; may extend to 10 weeks

Symptoms:
- Fits of numerous, rapid coughs followed by "whoop" sound
- Vomiting and exhaustion after coughing fits (called paroxysms)

Recovery: Stage 3
Last about 2 to 3 weeks; susceptible to other respiratory infections for many months

Recovery is gradual. Coughing lessens but fits of coughing may return.

cdc.gov/whoopingcough

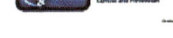

U.S. Department of
Health and Human Services
Centers for Disease
Control and Prevention

Fig. 2.29 Whooping cough's three-stage progression. (Picture Source: https://www.cdc.gov. CDC)

paroxysmal attacks occur more frequently at night (averaging 15 per 24 h) and afflicted infants and young children may become critically distressed and cyanotic. Vomiting and exhaustion may follow a spell of coughing, but between attacks the person generally appears quite well.
• Recovery is gradual in the convalescent stage, with coughing slowly subsiding over several weeks to months.

Whooping cough can result in serious complications, most commonly in babies and young children, with approximately one-third of infants under 1 year of age needing hospitalization. Among hospitalized infants, the most frequent cause of pertussis-related deaths is a secondary bacterial pneumonia. Neurological complications such as convulsions or encephalopathy are also of significant concern (possibly resulting from the hypoxia of coughing or the pertussis toxin), as are a cough-related pneumothorax, subdural hematoma, and hernia. Many less serious complications such as otitis media, anorexia, and dehydration may also occur. Approximately 1% of hospitalized pertussis-afflicted infants die from one or more associated complications [122, 123].

The diagnosis of whooping cough is principally based on clinical presentation coupled with culture of exudate from the posterior nasopharynx for the infecting organism. Ancillary tests include polymerase chain reaction (PCR) and serological tests, which may prove helpful in some cases where the diagnosis is unclear [123].

Treatment of pertussis is centered on supportive care. If administered early in the course of the infection (catarrhal stage), antibiotics (azithromycin, clarithromycin, and erythromycin) may be of therapeutic value and are helpful in decreasing contagion by eradicating bacteria in the secretions [123, 124].

****

There is no known animal or insect reservoir of *Bordetella pertussis* bacterium other than humans, which is passed from person-to-person with a communicable infection rate approaching 80% among susceptible (unvaccinated) household contacts [123]. Active infection does not afford lasting immunity so periodic vaccine immunization is required for prophylactic protection against the disease.

A whole-cell pertussis vaccine (suspensions of whole bacteria that have been killed) became widely available in the USA in the 1940s, and in 1948 the vaccine was combined with tetanus and diphtheria toxoid to form the ubiquitous DTP (or DTwP) vaccine. Concerns over safety and adverse side effects led to the development of a more purified acellular vaccine containing inactivated pertussis toxin and other antigenic bacterial components, which proved to be less reactogenic although of somewhat lower efficacy and shorter immunogenicity [123, 125].

Combined with the tetanus and diphtheria toxoid, the acellular vaccine is known as DTaP, with "aP" standing for "acellular pertussis." Approved in 1991 and put into universal use in 1997, the original DTP whole-cell vaccine is no longer licensed in the USA. The recommended/allocated constituent dosing strengths (amounts) within the current combination vaccine vary according to the recipient's age and primary v. booster status [123].

****

During the early years of the twentieth century, the morbidity and mortality associated with pertussis infections were staggering, particularly among young children. Between 1940 and 1945, more than 1 million pertussis cases were reported, averaging 17,500 cases per year, according to CDC data [123]. Following the introduction of the whole-cell vaccine, reported cases declined to 15,000 in 1960, 5000 in 1970, and approximately 2900 cases per year in the period between 1980 and 1990 [123].

In subsequent years, the reported incidence of pertussis cases has been on the rise in the USA (and throughout the world) with several epidemic outbreaks observed since the early 2000s [123]. Multiple factors are possibly at play. Heightened recognition and reporting of cases may be artificially enhancing incidence data. However, the transitioning to the acellular vaccines in the 1990s, with their lack of long-term immunity, appears to be of principal and paramount importance [123, 127].

New preventive strategies with recommendations for more frequent booster doses, new and improved vaccines, and vaccine hesitancy abatement/education may all be of importance in stemming the resurgent tide of this dreadful disease [126].

Mumps (*Parotitis*)

Once a common disease of childhood, many of today's physicians have never encountered a case of mumps, thanks to the vaccination program introduced in the USA in 1967. Unfortunately, like so many other infectious diseases, cases are on the rise, likely due to waning vaccine immunity among other factors [128, 129].

Mumps is a contagious viral illness caused by a paramyxovirus of the *Rubulavirus* family (Fig. 2.30), which is spread person-to-person through direct contact with saliva, or through respiratory droplets expelled during talking, coughing, or sneezing from an infected individual [128].

After an incubation period averaging 16–18 days, the mumps virus typically affects one or both parotid salivary glands, causing a telltale swelling in the cheek and jaw area (Fig. 2.31). The swelling usually peaks over 1–3 days, followed by gradual subsidence over an ensuing week. Nonspecific prodromal symptoms of fever, headache, myalgia, and weakness generally precede parotitis by several days [128, 130].

Although most people recover uneventfully from mumps infections within a couple of weeks from the onset of symptoms, a small percentage of persons suffer significant complications, most commonly in those infected as adolescents or adults. Inflammation of the ovaries (oophoritis), breasts (mastitis), and testicles (orchitis) generally resolves without long-term sequelae, but testicular atrophy and hypofertility may result. Pancreatitis, deafness, meningitis, and encephalitis are recognized complications but are reported in under 1% of cases [128, 130].

The diagnosis of mumps is principally based on the patient's clinical presentation. Real-time polymerase chain reaction (RT-PCR) and viral cultures are helpful in confirming the diagnosis, as is IgM serology in some cases. Treatment is supportive and vaccination with the MMR vaccine is safe and effective [128, 130].

****

Fig. 2.30 Graphical
representation of the
mumps virus. (Picture
Source: http://phil.cdc.gov.
CDC: Public Health Image
Library)

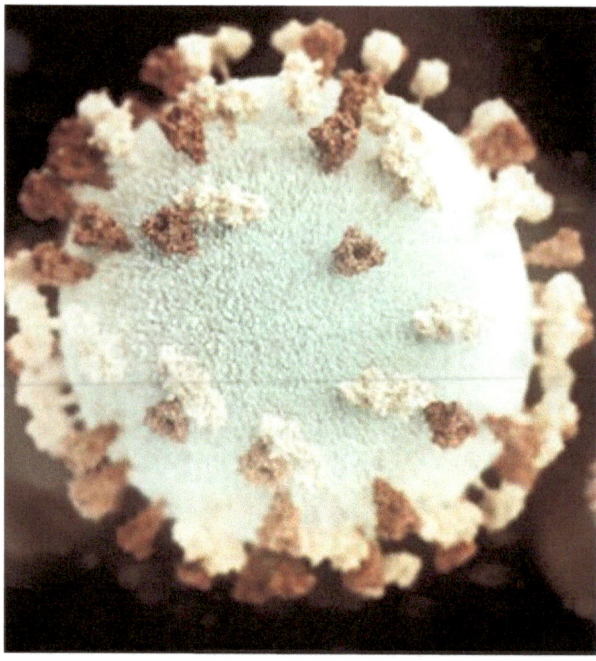

Fig. 2.31 Child with a
mumps infection and
characteristic parotitis.
(Picture Source: http://phil.
cdc.gov. CDC: Public
Health Image Library)

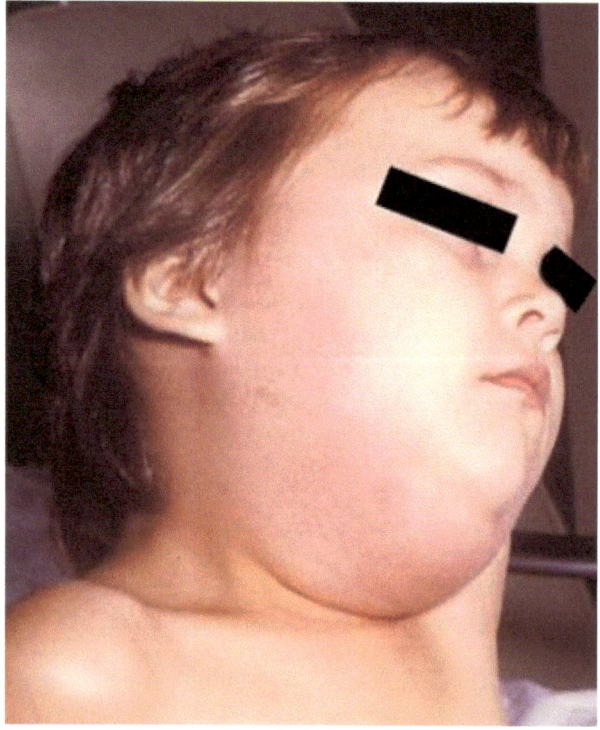

The live-attenuated mumps vaccine currently approved for use in the USA was developed by the prodigious Merck vaccinologist, Maurice Hillman (1919–2005), and licensed for use in 1967 [129, 131]. The seed virus used in the vaccine was isolated from Hillman's five-year-old daughter when she was ill with mumps and is still in use in the mumps vaccine today, referred to as the "Jeryl Lynn" strain.

Hillman is the credited developer of more than 40 vaccines, including those used to protect against measles, mumps, rubella, *Haemophilus influenzae* type b, hepatitis A, hepatitis B, and chickenpox [131, 132]. In 1971, the mumps vaccine was licensed in the USA in combination with the measles and rubella vaccines to form the ubiquitous MMR vaccine, updated with an improved rubella component in 1979 [129, 133].

An unfortunate setback in vaccine history was the dishonest and discredited 1998 publication by Andrew J. Wakefield in *The Lancet*, linking the MMR vaccine to autism (see the **Measles** section). Leading to a sharp drop in vaccination rates and catalyzing the anti-vaccination movement, the study is considered to be one of the most damaging pieces of medical literature in modern medicine [129].

Be that as it may, the recommended two-dose MMR vaccine protocol initiated in 1967 dramatically reduced the incidence of mumps in the USA. Infection rates were lowered by 99% from the pre-vaccine era, with just a few hundred reported cases per year until the early 2000s, according to CDC data [128]. However, since 2006 there has been an uptick of cases, with outbreaks ranging from a few hundred to several thousand cases, a majority occurring in fully vaccinated individuals living in close-contact settings [128].

Research studies implicate a waning vaccine-derived immunity as responsible for the case resurgence, suggesting that an additional booster dose may be indicated for individuals over 18 years of age [129]. Although most industrialized nations include mumps-containing vaccines as part of their national immunization programs, the 2007 WHO position statement states that *"Based on mortality and disease burden, WHO considers measles control and the prevention of congenital rubella syndrome to be higher priorities than the control of mumps* [133]," suggesting an unlikelihood referable to any new global mumps-specific vaccination initiative in the near future.

Meningitis (*Spinal Meningitis*)

Meningitis is an infection and/or inflammation of the membranes surrounding the brain and spinal cord (meninges), commonly caused by several species of bacteria—principally *Neisseria meningitidis* (meningococcus), *Streptococcus pneumonia* (pneumococcus), *Haemophilus influenzae,* and *Streptococcus agalactiae* (group B streptococcus). Viruses (enteroviruses, measles, mumps), fungi (*Coccidioides*), and the so-called brain eating ameba parasite (*Naegleria fowleri*) are less common causes. Rarely, drugs and other non-infective inflammatory conditions can cause meningitis [134, 135].

An ancient disease, likely first described by Hippocrates (460–370 BCE), the term "meningitis" was coined in the 1800s by French and English physicians, combining the anatomic term for the lining of the brain (meninges) with the suffix "itis," suggesting inflammation. Outbreaks of meningitis around the world were identified in the early 1800s, but it was not until 1887 that Austrian bacteriologist Anton Weichselbaum (1845–1920) isolated the bacterium *Diplococcus intracellularis meningitides* (renamed *Neisseria meningitides* in 1901) from the cerebrospinal fluid of patients diagnosed with bacterial meningitis. In 1890, Heinrich Quincke (1842–1922) introduced the lumbar spinal puncture to identify the causative organism, which remains the principal diagnostic tool in use today [136].

Bacterial meningitis is the most common and dangerous type of meningitis, with death ensuing within 24 h following the onset of symptoms in some cases. Common symptoms include a stiff neck, fever, rash, headache, nausea and vomiting, photophobia, and an altered mental status. Babies may become lethargic, irritable or inconsolable, floppy or stiff, and difficult to arouse. Worldwide, around 1 in 6 person's die and 1 in 5 persons have severe complications including septicemia, hearing or vision loss, seizures, cognitive impairment, and limb loss or weakness (Fig. 2.32) following bacterial meningitis infections [134, 135].

Most of the bacteria and viruses that cause meningitis are carried in the nose and throat and are spread by respiratory droplets or throat secretions. Group B streptococcus organisms are also carried in the gut or vagina and may infect a newborn during childbirth. Fungus-laden environmental dust is potentially causative if inhaled (principally cryptococcus) and ameba may be encountered in contaminated swimming or drinking water, commonly gaining entry through the nose.

With respect to bacterial meningitis, newborns are at greatest risk from group B streptococcus, young children from meningococcus, pneumococcus, and

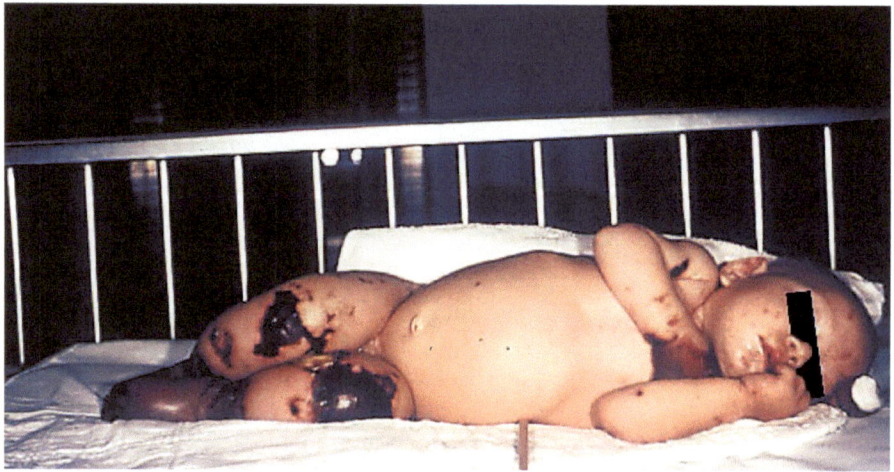

Fig. 2.32 Limb gangrene in infant due to meningococcemia. (Picture Source: https://www.cdc.gov. CDC: Public Health Image Library)

Haemophilus influenzae, adolescents and young adults from meningococcus, and the elderly from pneumococcus [134]. The highest burden of disease is in the sub-Saharan Africa "meningitis belt," with outbreaks of meningococcal and pneumococcal meningitis most common [134, 137].

The diagnosis of meningitis is based on clinical presentation coupled with a lumbar spinal tap to identify the causative organism by microscopic examination and culture of the withdrawn spinal fluid. Blood cultures are also helpful in determining the infecting organism in the presence of systemic infection (sepsis). Antigen/antibody tests and/or polymerase chain reaction (PCR) tests of blood samples provide rapid diagnostic tests, as well [134, 135].

Treatment is an unqualified medical emergency with organism-specific antibiotics (or antifungal or anti-parasitic medications) coupled with supportive care, with the outcome frequently determined by the rapidity of diagnosis and initiation of treatment. Antiviral drugs may be administered in some cases. Antibiotic prophylaxis is often recommended for persons in close (household) contact with an infected person with bacterial meningitis, particularly those with meningococcal disease [134].

Prior to the availability of antibiotics, anti-meningococcal antibody serum, derived from infected horses or from persons who had recovered from meningococcal disease, was used to treat meningococcal meningitis and provide prophylactic protection to persons at exposure risk. The antibiotic era began in the 1930s when Sara Branham (1888–1962) found that the newly introduced sulfonamides effectively treated meningococcus. The advent of penicillin availability in the early 1940s began the modern antibiotic era, with several current-generation antibiotics used to treat all varieties of bacterial meningitis [136].

****

Vaccines against the common types of bacterial meningitis have been available for a number of years, as well as the common causes of viral meningitis (measles, mumps, etc.), greatly decreasing the burden of disease in the USA and other developed countries [134, 138].

Meningococcus bacteria exhibit multiple serotypes, necessitating different vaccines targeting the most common infective varieties. Currently, there are three quadrivalent conjugate vaccines against serogroups A, C, W, and Y (*MenACWY*) and two recombinant serogroup B vaccines (*MenB*) approved for use in the USA. These are selectively recommended by the CDC for different age groups and persons within various "at risk" categories [139]. All have a high initial protective efficacy but, like many other vaccines, tend to wane in their protective capability with time [139]. The vaccines are safe, with mild post-vaccination symptoms (sore injection site, low-grade fever, muscle or joint pain, fatigue, headache, etc.) being relatively common [134, 136, 139].

Within the general age-group susceptibilities mentioned previously are additional risk factors for meningitis, most notably for meningococcal infections. Among other factors, people living in close proximity are at higher risk, specifically those living in overcrowded households or residing in student or military institutions where communal housing, common dining facilities, and shared food and drinks are the norm [140].

Currently, only a quadrivalent vaccine (*MenACWY*) is recommended for 11- to 12-year-olds (followed by a suggested booster at age 16) as part of the routine pediatric vaccination schedule, leaving serogroup B as the leading cause of meningococcal meningitis in young adults [141]. Among college students, meningococcus B is responsible for 100% of the outbreaks that have occurred on college campuses since 2009, causing 43 infections and 3 deaths [140]. As such, the CDC has advised that teens and young adults consider extending their immunization protection with a *MenB* vaccine if they fall within a high-risk group or are residing in conditions where an outbreak has occurred or seems likely [141].

Additionally, the CDC has reported that there is currently (2021–2023) a serogroup C meningococcal disease outbreak in Florida affecting a wide range of people, but principally gay and bisexual men [142]. The CDC has recommended that gay and bisexual men get a *MenACWY* vaccine if they live in Florida or are traveling to Florida. Around half of the cases are among Hispanic men and some are living with HIV [142].

References

1918 Pandemic Influenza

1. Barry JM. The great influenza: the epic story of the deadliest plague in history. New York: Penguin Books; 2005.
2. Taubenberger JK, Morens DM. 1918 influenza: the mother of all pandemics. Emerg Infect Dis. 2006;12(1):15–22. https://www.ncbi.nlm.nih.gov.
3. Royde-Smith JG. Casualties of World War I: killed wounded and missing. Encyclopedia Britannica; 2023. https://www.britannica.com.
4. Thompson G. American military operations and casualties in 1917-18. University of Kansas Medical Center; 2023. https://www.kumc.edu.
5. Weaver PC, Van Bergen L. Death from 1918 pandemic influenza during the first world war: a perspective from personal and anecdotal evidence. Influenza Other Respir Viruses. 2014;8(5):538–46. https://www.ncbi.nlm.nih.gov.
6. Roos R. Scientists recreate 1918 flu virus, see parallels with H5N1. Center for Infectious Disease Research and Policy (CIDRAP) News; 2005. https://www.cidrap.umn.edu.
7. Litzinger M. The 1918-1919 influenza pandemic as covered in *The JI*. The American Association of Immunologists—History of the JI; 2012. https://www.aai.org.
8. Barry JM. How the horrific 1918 flu spread across America. Smithsonian Magazine. 2017. https://www.smithsonianmag.com.
9. CDC. 1918 pandemic influenza: three waves. Centers for Disease Control and Prevention; 2018. https://www.cdc.gov.
10. Arnold C. Pandemic 1918: eyewitness accounts from the greatest medical holocaust in modern history. New York: St. Martin's Griffin; 2020.
11. Fajgenbaum DC, June CH. Cytokine storm. N Engl J Med. 2020;383(23):2255–73. https://www.ncbi.nlm.nih.gov.

12. Aanmoen O. The king whose illness led to the naming of a pandemic. Royal Central; 2020. https://royalcentra.com.uk.
13. CDC. Influenza (flu): 2022-2023 U.S. flu season: preliminary in-season burden estimates. Centers for Disease Control and Prevention; 2023. https://www.cdc.gov.

Hansen's Disease

14. Santacroce L, Del Prete R, Charitos IA, Bottalico L. *Mycobacterium leprae*: a histological study on the origins of leprosy and its social stigma. Infez Med. 2021;29(4):623–32. https://www.ncbi.nlm.nih.gov.
15. The Leprosy Mission. Leprosy in the Bible. The Leprosy Mission International; 2022. https://www.leprosymission.org.
16. Nardell EA. Leprosy. Merck Manual: professional version. 2022. https://www.merckmanuals.com.
17. CDC. Hansen's disease (leprosy): transmission. Centers for Disease Control and Prevention; 2017. https://www.cdc.gov.
18. WHO. Leprosy. World Health Organization; 2022. https://www.who.int.
19. Creative Biolabs. *Mycobacterium leprae* vaccines. Creative Biolabs; 2022. https://www.creative-biolabs.com.
20. Duthie MS, Pena MT, Ebenezer GJ, et al. LepVax, a defined subunit vaccine that provides effective pre-exposure and post-exposure prophylaxis of *M. leprae* infection. NPI Vacc. 2018;3:12. https://www.nature.com.
21. CDC. Hansen's disease (leprosy). Centers for Disease Control and Prevention; 2021. https://www.cdc.gov.
22. Truman RW, Singh P, Sharma R, et al. Probable zoonotic leprosy in the southern United States. N Engl J Med. 2011;364(17):1626–33. https://www.ncbi.nlm.nih.gov.
23. Wong A. When the last patient dies. The Atlantic. 2015. https://www.theatlantic.com.
24. Penikese Island School. History of Penikese Island. Penikese Island School, Inc.; 2022. https://www.penikese.org.
25. ILA. History of leprosy: The United States of America. International Leprosy Association; 2022. https://leprosyhistory.org.
26. Gaudlip A. Revisiting Louisiana's Medical legacy: The National Leprosarium in Carville. Preservation Resource Center of New Orleans; 2020. https://prcno.org.
27. Nature Publishing Group. Treatment of leprosy. Nature. 1932;130:234. https://www.nature.com.
28. HRSA. History of the National Hansen's Disease (Leprosy) Program: Carville Hospital timeline. Health Resources & Services Administration; 2018. https://www.hrsa.gov.

Smallpox

29. Ochmann S, Roser M. Smallpox. Our world in data. 2018. https://www.ourworldindata.org/smallpox.
30. AMNH. Smallpox: lessons from the past. American Museum of Natural History; 2022. https://www.amnh.org.
31. WHO. History of smallpox vaccinations. World Health Organization; 2022. https://www.who.int.
32. CDC. Smallpox. Centers for Disease Control and Prevention; 2016. https://www.cdc.gov.
33. Muhlemann B, Vinner L, Sikora M, et al. Diverse variola virus (smallpox) strains were widespread in northern Europe in the Viking Age. Science. 2020;369:6502. https://www.science.org.

34. CDC. History of smallpox. Centers for Disease Control and Prevention; 2021. https://www.cdc.gov.
35. Greenspan J. The rise and fall of smallpox. History. 2020. https://www.history.com.
36. Hasselgren P-O. The smallpox epidemics in America in the 1700s and the role of the surgeons: lessons to be learned during the global outbreak of COVID-19. World J Surg. 2020;44(9):2837–41. https://www.ncbi.nlm.nih.gov.
37. Archives and Records Management. On this day in 1721, Dr. Zabdiel Boylston inoculates his son against smallpox. City of Boston Archives and Records Management; 2017. https://www.boston.gov.
38. Boylston A, Williams AE. Zabdiel Boylston's evaluation of inoculation against smallpox. J R Soc Med. 2008;101(9):476–7. https://www.ncbi.nlm.nih.gov.
39. Roos D. How crude smallpox inoculations helped George Washington win the war. History. 2020. https://www.history.com.
40. Fenn E. The great smallpox epidemic. History Today. 2003;53:8. https://www.historytoday.com.
41. The Jenner Institute. About Edward Jenner. The Jenner Institute; 2023. https://www.jenner.ac.uk.
42. Charleston LJ. Smallpox and the photos anti-vaxxers don't want you to see. Lifestyle. 2019. https://www.nzhearld.co.nz.
43. CDC. Smallpox bioterrorism. Centers for Disease Control and Prevention; 2016. https://www.cdc.gov.
44. WHO. Monkeypox. World Health Organization; 2022. https://www.who.int.
45. NIH. Smallpox. NIH: National Institute of Allergy and Infectious Diseases; 2014. https://www.niaid.nih.gov.

Rubeola

46. CDC. Measles (rubella): for healthcare workers. Centers for Disease Control and Prevention; 2020. https://www.cdc.gov.
47. NFID. Measles. National Foundation for Infectious Diseases; 2022. https://www.nfid.org.
48. WHO. Measles. World Health Organization; 2019. https://www.who.int.
49. Mayo Clinic. Measles. Mayo Clinic; 2022. https://www.mayoclinic.org.
50. WHO. History of the measles vaccine: one of the most contagious diseases. World Health Organization; 2023. https://www.who.int.
51. Katz SL, John F. Enders and measles virus vaccine—reminiscence. Curr Top Microbiol Immunol. 2009;329:3–11. https://pubmed.ncbi.nlm.nih.gov.
52. Tulchinsky TH. Maurice Hilleman: creator of vaccines that changed the world. Case Studies in Public Health; 2018. https://www.ncbi.nlm.nih.gov.
53. Wakefield AJ, Murch SH, Anthony A, et al. Ileal-lymphoid-nodular hyperplasia, non-specific colitis, and pervasive developmental disorder in children. The Lancet. 1998;351:637–41. https://www.thelancet.com.
54. Nature Medicine. A timeline of the Wakefield retraction. Nat Med. 2010;16:248. https://nature.com.
55. Eggertson L. Lancet retracts 12-year-old article linking autism to MMR vaccines. CMAJ. 2010;182(4):E199–200. https://www.ncbi.nlm.nih.gov.
56. CDC. Measles cases and outbreaks. Centers for Disease Control and Prevention; 2023. https://www.cdc.gov.
57. CDC. Global measles outbreaks. Centers for Disease Control and Prevention; 2023. https://www.cdc.gov.
58. Phadke VK, Bednarczyk RA, Omer SB. Vaccine refusal and measles outbreaks in the US. JAMA. 2020;324(13):1344–5. https://jamanetwork.com.

59. Gardner L, Dong E, Khan K, et al. Persistence of US measles risk due to vaccine hesitancy and outbreaks abroad. The Lancet. 2020;20(10):1114–5. https://www.thelancet.com.
60. Iacobucci G. Measles is now "an imminent threat" globally, WHO and CDC warn. BMJ. 2022;379:2844. https://www.bmj.com.
61. WHO. Global measles threat continues to grow as another year passes with millions of children unvaccinated. World Health Organization; 2023. https://www.who.int.

Rubella

62. NCIRD. Rubella in the U.S. National Center for Immunization and Respiratory Diseases (NCIRD). Division of Viral Diseases; 2020. https://www.cdc.gov.
63. History of Vaccines. Rubella (German measles). The College of Physicians of Philadelphia; 2023. https://historyofvaccines.org.
64. Stanley A, Plotkin MD; NFID. Recipient of the 2009 Maxwell Finland Award for Scientific Achievement. National Foundation for Infectious Diseases; 2023. https://www.nfid.org.
65. Tulchinsky TH. Maurice Hilleman: creator of vaccines that changed the world. Case Studies in Public Health; 2018. https://www.ncbi.nlm.nih.gov.
66. WHO. Rubella. World Health Organization; 2019. https://www.who.int.
67. Shukla S, Maraqa NF. Congenital rubella. NCBI Bookshelf: National Library of Medicine, National Institutes of Health; 2022. http://www.ncbi.nlm.nih.gov.
68. CDC. Pregnancy and rubella. Centers for Disease Control and Prevention; 2020. https://www.cdc.gov.

Tuberculosis

69. Gradmann C. Robert Koch and the white death: from tuberculosis to tuberculin. Microbes Infect. 2006;8(1):294–301. https://pubmed.ncbi.nlm.nih.gov.
70. CDC. Historical perspectives centennial: Koch's discovery of the tubercle bacillus. MMWR. 1982;31(10):121–3. https://www.cdc.gov.
71. CDC. Tuberculosis (TB): history of world TB day. Centers for Disease Control and Prevention, Division of Tuberculosis Elimination; 2023. https://www.cdc.gov.
72. Daniel TM. The history of tuberculosis. J Resp Med. 2006;100(11):1862–70. https://www.sciencedirect.com.
73. CDC. Tuberculosis (TB): basic TB facts. Centers for Disease Control and Prevention; 2022. https://www.cdc.gov.
74. Bandari J, Thada PK. Scrofula. NCBI Bookshelf; 2022. https://www.ncbi.nlm.nih.gov.
75. Al Ubaidi BA. The radiological diagnosis of pulmonary tuberculosis (TB) in primary care. J Fam Med Dis Prev. 2018;4(1):73. https://www.clinmedjournals.org.
76. Harding F. Florence Seibert. The Lancet. 2017;5(4):255–6. https://www.thelancet.com.
77. CDC. Tuberculosis (TB): testing for TB infection. Centers for Disease Control and Prevention; 2022. https://www.cdc.gov.
78. Waters M, Tadi P. Streptomycin. NCBI Bookshelf; 2022. https://www.ncbi.nlm.nih.gov.
79. WHO. BCG vaccine. World Health Organization; 2023. https://www.who.int.
80. Okafor CN, Rewane A, Momodu II. Bacillus Calmette Guerin. NCBI Bookshelf; 2022. https://www.ncbi.nlm.nih.gov.
81. Vohra S, Dhaliwai HS. Miliary tuberculosis. NCBI Bookshelf; 2022. https://www.ncbi.nlm.nih.gov.
82. Kanabus A. Sanatorium—from the first to the last. Information about tuberculosis. GHE; 2022. www.tbfacts.org.

83. Van Crevel R, Hill PC. Plombage—an overview. In: Infectious diseases. 4th ed. Amsterdam: Elsevier; 2017. https://www.sciencedirect.com.
84. Murray JF, Schraufnagel DE, Hopewell PE. Treatment of tuberculosis. a historical perspective. Ann Am Thorac Soc. 2015;12(12):1749–59. https://www.atsjournals.org.
85. ALS. Christmas Seals history. American Lung Association; 2023. https://www.lung.org.
86. Dawson JJY, Devadatta S, Fox W, et al. A 5-year study of patients with pulmonary tuberculosis in a concurrent comparison of home and sanatorium treatment for one year with isoniazid and PAS. Bull World Health Organ. 1966;34(4):533–51. https://www.ncbi.nlm.nih.gov.
87. Kanabus A. History of tuberculosis (TB)—world history, start of TB, then through the centuries. Information About Tuberculosis: GHE; 2022. https://www.tbfacts.org.
88. Somocurcio JG, Sotomayor A, Shin S, et al. Surgery for patients with drug-resistant tuberculosis: report of 121 cases receiving community-based treatment in Lima, Peru. Thorax. 2007;62(5):416–21. https://www.ncbi.nlm.nih.gov.
89. WHO. Tuberculosis. World Health Organization; 2022. https://www.who.int.
90. WHO. Tuberculosis deaths and disease increase during the Covid-19 pandemic. World Health Organization; 2022. https://www.who.int.
91. CDC. Global health: tuberculosis. Centers for Disease Control and Prevention; 2022. https://www.cdc.gov.
92. WHO. Tuberculosis. World Health Organization; 2023. https://www.who.int.
93. UN News. New global action pledge to end TB by 2030. United Nations News; 2023. https://news.un.org.

Group A Streptococcal Disease

94. ASM. Scarlet fever: a deadly history and how it prevails. American Society of Microbiology; 2023. https://asm.org.
95. CDC. Group A streptococcal (GAS) disease. Centers for Disease Control and Prevention; 2022. https://www.cdc.gov.
96. Ferretti J, Köhler W. History of streptococcal research. NCBI Bookshelf: National Library of Medicine, National Institutes of Health; 2016. https://www.ncbi.nlm.nih.gov.
97. CDC. Rheumatic fever: all you need to know. Centers for Disease Control and Prevention; 2022. https://www.cdc.gov.
98. Weinberg GA. Rheumatic fever. Merck Manual: consumer version. 2022. https://www.merckmanuals.com.

Varicella

99. CDC. Chickenpox (varicella). National Center for Immunization and Respiratory Diseases (NCIRD), Division of Viral Diseases; 2021. https://www.cdc.gov.
100. Ayoade F, Kumar S. Varicella zoster (chickenpox). NCBI Bookshelf: National Library of Medicine, National Institutes of Health; 2022. https://www.ncbi.nlm.nih.gov.
101. WHO. Varicella. World Health Organization; 2023. https://www.who.int.
102. Bracho-Sanchez E. Chickenpox parties and natural immunity: your questions answered. CNN Health; 2019. https://www.cnn.com.
103. Marin M, Seward JF, Gershon AA. 25 Years of varicella vaccination in the United States. J Infect Dis. 2022;226(4):375–9. https://academic.oup.com.
104. Kota V Grella MJ. Varicella (chickenpox) vaccine. NCBI Bookshelf: National Library of Medicine, National Institutes of Health; 2023. https://www.ncbi.nlm.nih.gov.
105. CDC. MMRV (measles, mumps, rubella & varicella) VIS. Centers for Disease Control and Prevention; 2021. https://www.cdc.gov.

106. Mayo Clinic. Reye's syndrome. Mayo Clinic; 2023. https://www.mayoclinic.org.
107. CDC. Shingles (herpes zoster). National Center for Immunization and Respiratory Diseases (NCIRD), Division of Viral Diseases; 2019. https://www.cdc.gov.
108. MedlinePlus. Shingles. MedlinePlus: National Institutes of Health/National Library of Medicine; 2023. https://medlineplus.gov.
109. CDC. Shingles vaccination: what everyone should know about the shingles vaccine (Shingrix). Centers for Disease Control and Prevention; 2022. https://www.cdc.gov.
110. Cleveland Clinic. Shingles. Cleveland Clinic; 2022. https://my.clevelandclinic.org.

Diphtheria

111. History of Vaccines/College of Physicians of Philadelphia. Diphtheria: *Corynebacterium diphtheriae*. College of Physicians of Philadelphia; 2023. https://historyofvaccines.org.
112. Baumgartner L. Edwin Klebs—a centennial note. N Engl J Med. 1935;213:60–3. https://www.nejm.org.
113. CDC. Diphtheria. Centers for Disease Control and Prevention; 2022. https://www.cdc.gov.
114. Berih A. Cutaneous *Corynebacterium diphtheriae*: a traveler's disease. Can J Infect Dis. 1995;6(3):150–2. https://www.ncbi.nlm.nih.gov.
115. CDC. Diphtheria: clinical information. Centers for Disease Control and Prevention; 2022. https://www.cdc.gov.
116. Dittrick Medical History Center. Deadly diphtheria: the children's plague. Dittrick Medical History Center; 2017. https://artsci.case.edu/dittrick.
117. Acosta AM, Moro PL, Hariri S, et al. Diphtheria. In: "The Pink Book". 14th ed. Atlanta: Centers for Disease Control and Prevention; 2021. https://www.cdc.gov.
118. Meinikov VG, Berger A, Sing A. Detection of diphtheria toxin production by toxigenic corynebacteria using an optimized Elek test. Infection. 2022;50(6):1591–5. https://www.ncbi.nlm.nih.gov.
119. Bisgard KM, Hardy IR, Popovic T, et al. Respiratory diphtheria in the United States, 1980 through 1995. Am J Public Health. 1998;88(5):787–91. https://www.ncbi.nlm.nih.gov.
120. PAHO/WHO. Diphtheria. Pan American Health Organization/World Health Organization; 2022. https://www.paho.org.
121. Anderson P, Solomon M, Ramlatchan S, et al. Diphtheria re-emerges in the unimmunized. IDCases. 2021;23:e01020. https://www.ncbi.nlm.nih.gov.

Pertussis

122. CDC. Pertussis (whooping cough): signs and symptoms. Centers for Disease Control and Prevention; 2022. https://www.cdc.gov.
123. Havers FP, Moro PL, Hariri S, et al. Pertussis. In: "The Pink Book". 14th ed. Centers for Disease Control and Prevention; 2021. https://www.cdc.gov.
124. History of Vaccines/College of Physicians of Philadelphia. Pertussis (whooping cough). College of Physicians of Philadelphia; 2022. https://historyofvaccines.org.
125. Alghounaim M, Alsaffar Z, Alfrajj A, et al. Whole-cell and acellular pertussis vaccine: reflections on efficacy. Med Princ Pract. 2022;31(4):313–21. https://karger.com.
126. Kuchar E, Karlikowska-Skwarnik M, Han S, et al. Pertussis: history of the disease and current prevention failure. Adv Exp Med Biol. 2016;934:77–82. https://pubmed.ncbi.nlm.nih.gov.
127. Cherry JD. The history of pertussis (whooping cough); 1906-2015: facts, myths, and misconceptions. Curr Epidemiol Rep. 2015;2:120–30. https://link.springer.com.

Mumps

128. CDC. Mumps: for health care professionals. Centers for Disease Control and Prevention; 2021. https://www.cdc.gov.
129. Gardner E. Tracing the story of mumps: a timeline. Pharmaceutical Technology. 2018. https://www.pharmaceutical-technology.com.
130. Cleveland Clinic. Mumps. Cleveland Clinic; 2022. https://my.clevelandclinic.org.
131. Newman L. Maurice Hilleman. BMJ. 2005;330:7498. https://www.ncbi.nlm.nih.gov.
132. Dove A. Maurice Hilleman. Nat Med. 2005;11:S2. https://www.nature.com.
133. WHO. Mumps virus vaccines: WHO position paper, 2007. World Health Organization. Wkly Epidemiol Rec. 2007;82:7. https://www.who.int.

Meningitis

134. WHO. Meningitis. World Health Organization; 2023. https://www.who.int.
135. Cleveland Clinic. Meningitis. Cleveland Clinic; 2022.; https://my.clevelandclinic.org.
136. Edwards H. The history of meningitis. Meningitis Research Foundation; 2020. https://www.meningitis.org.
137. CDC. Meningococcal disease: meningococcal disease in other countries. Centers for Disease Control and Prevention; 2022. https://www.cdc.gov.
138. CDC. Meningococcal disease: clinical information. Centers for Disease Control and Prevention; 2022. https://www.cdc.gov.
139. Mbaeyi S, Duffy J, McNamara LA. Meningococcal disease. In: "The Pink Book". 14th ed. Centers for Disease Control and Prevention; 2021. https://www.cdc.gov.
140. Chung GS, Hutton DW. Epidemiological impact and cost-effectiveness of universal meningitis B vaccination among college students prior to college entry. PLoS One. 2020;15(10):e0239926. https://www.ncbi.nlm.nih.gov.
141. CDC. Meningococcal disease: meningococcal vaccination. Centers for Disease Control and Prevention; 2022. https://www.cdc.gov.
142. CDC. Meningococcal disease: meningococcal disease outbreak among gay, bisexual men in Florida, 2021-2023. Centers for Disease Control and Prevention; 2022. https://www.cdc.gov.

Chapter 3
Vector-Borne/Zoonotic Diseases

Abstract Zoonotic diseases are spread from animals to humans by direct contact with the infected animal (or its bodily fluids), ingesting infected meat or animal-contaminated food or water, or by an intermediary vector ("vector-borne") such as mosquitoes, fleas, lice and ticks. Some vector-borne diseases have been globally eradicated. Others are currently rare in the United States while continuing to afflict large segments of the global population. A few seem to be increasing in incidence, in part due to global warming and the associated prolongation of breeding periods and the spread of viable insect habitat. Additionally, ever-increasing insecticide resistance has hampered global efforts in controlling mosquitoes and other disease-transmitting vectors.

The vector-borne/zoonotic diseases discussed in this chapter, along with their historical names and monikers, are: Plague (*Bubonic Plague, Black Death*), Yellow Fever (*Bronze John, Yellow Jack*), Typhus (*Ship Fever, Jail Fever*), Malaria (*Swamp Fever, Ague, Congestive Fever*), Dengue (*Breakbone Fever, Seven-day Fever*), Rabies, Rocky Mountain Spotted Fever (*Black Measles*).

Plague (*Bubonic Plague, Black Death*)

Perhaps the deadliest disease of all time, plague is now known to be caused by the bacterium *Yersinia pestis*, a zoonotic bacillus typically found in rats and other small mammals. Generally transmitted between animals and humans by the bite of infected fleas, direct contact with infected tissues (animal or human) or inhalation of infected respiratory droplets are also modes of transmission, albeit less common.[1]

---

[1] The reader might enjoy the historical novel by Geraldine Brooks titled *Year of Wonders: A Novel of the Plague* (Viking Penguin, 2001). The book is inspired by the true story of the town of Eyam in rural England, during the plague of 1666.

Fig. 3.1 Citizens of
Tournai bury plague
victims. Pierart dou Tielt
1340–1360. (Picture
Source: https://en.
wickipedia.org. *Chronicles
of Gilles Li Muisis*
(1272–1352) Royal
Library of Belgium)

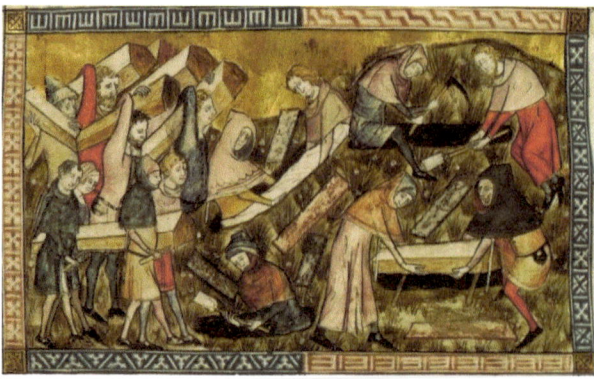

Principally of historical interest at this time, the epidemiological history of
plague is generally divided into three major pandemics, with multiple smaller outbreaks in intervening years [1].

The first was the "Justinian Plague" of 541–544, concentrated in North Africa
and the Middle East. The second is referred to as the "Black Death of 1347," with
millions of people affected throughout most of Europe during its years of peak
intensity (1347–1352), then lasting in sporadic outbreaks (e.g., The Great Plague of
London of 1665 to 1666) well into the eighteenth century (Fig. 3.1). The third outbreak, of somewhat lesser magnitude, is known as the "Third Pandemic of 1894."
Initially affecting port cities of China, it spread to Australia and the USA in limited
outbreaks and in larger numbers to India, waxing and waning throughout the world
over the ensuing five decades, killing millions [1].

The total estimated number of deaths associated with plague varies considerably from author to author; but, at minimum, the number is staggering—particularly relative to the world's population at the time, and certainly in the high
tens-of-millions, if not well over a hundred million [2].[2] Reporting in *Science* in
2020 [3], Lizzie Wade states that "In 1349, the Black Death killed about half of all
Londoners; from 1347 to 1351, it killed between 30% and 60% of all Europeans."

Regardless of the mode of transmission, plague was a horrendous way to die.
After a short incubation period, infected lymph nodes in the neck, axilla, and groin
typically swelled into large purulent black tumors (known as buboes), giving the
disease its signature moniker, *bubonic plague*. High fever, hematemesis (bloody
vomit), necrotic skin, and delirium frequently followed the initial infection. Death
by septicemic shock and multiple organ failure, referred to as *septicemic plague*,
occurred in 30–60% of bubonic plague victims. If the disease spread to the lungs,
known as *pneumonic plague*, the infection became directly transmissible by droplet
contagion and was universally fatal in the pre-antibiotic era [4].

---

[2]For a graphic comparison of mortality statistics associated with major pandemics throughout
recorded history (including COVID-19), the reader is referred to the web site produced by *The
Washington Post* in 2020 (https://www.washingtonpost.com/graphics/2020/local/retropolis/
coronavirus-deadliest-pandemics).

An understanding of disease etiology and transmission during the first two plague eras was non-existent by today's standards. The concept of a pathogenic organism was completely unknown. Prevailing thought regarded "bad air" as the source of most illnesses, as discussed in previous sections. Divine punishment for sins committed was an etiological theory embraced by many to explain the plague pandemics, leading to an uptick in religious zealots practicing self-flagellation as atonement for their sins [5]. Jews were commonly blamed for the spread of the Black Death and antisemitism intensified throughout Europe during plague pandemics. Violent mobs attacked many Jewish communities, killing thousands of Jews [6].

Effective treatment for plague victims was also non-existent in the Middle Ages. With no idea how to deal with the disease, physicians tried everything and anything [7]. Vinegar mixed with herbs was thought to be protective against disease, as were flaming torches and scented fumigants. Rubbing raw onions on buboes was believed to draw out toxins and combat miasmic ("bad air") spread of disease (Fig. 3.2).

Bloodletting, using a fleam (knife-like phlebotome) or leaches, to purge bad humors was a universal "cure-all." Live chickens, snake parts, urine, and raw feces applied to buboes and skin sores to contest evil humors were all tried. None worked and, by today's understanding, were likely detrimental. Wealthy individuals could afford to leave infected regions which, no doubt, was helpful in avoiding disease on

Fig. 3.2 Seventeenth century plague doctor: costumed to drive away evil spirits, with a long beak filled with fragrant herbs to combat miasmic air. Circa 1656. (Picture Source: https://www.worldhistory.org. The engraving was first published by Paul Fürst (1608–1666) in *Europas Sprung in die Neuzeit*, by Johannes Ebert)

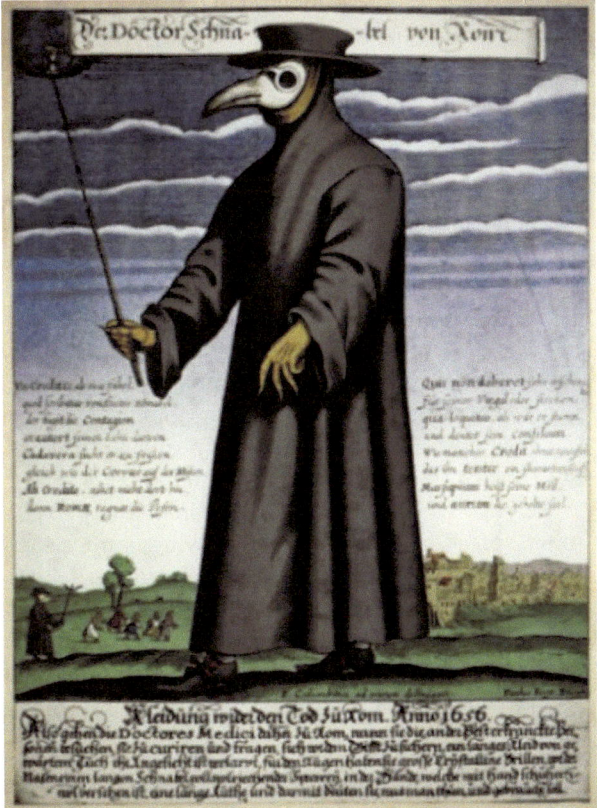

an individual basis. The quarantine of sick individuals, traveling visitors, and arriving ships, carried out by some communities, may also have limited the spread of disease.

****

The pandemic of 1894 reached America in 1900. Ships sailing from Hong Kong and Hawaii to San Francisco had plague aboard, possibly carried by Chinese immigrants but most assuredly by ship rats [8].

On March 6, 1900, Dr. Joseph Kinyoun (1860–1919) of the federal Marine Hospital Service (MHS), precursor to the modern U.S. Public Health Service, examined a bubo autopsy specimen from a deceased Chinese resident of Chinatown, San Francisco, who was suspected of dying from plague. Working from his laboratory on Angel Island in San Francisco Bay, Dr. Kinyoun—a prominent bacteriologist in his own right—identified and cultured the bacillus that was known to cause plague from the autopsy specimen, clinching the patient's diagnosis and formally marking the onset of San Francisco's plague epidemic.[3]

Several similar cases followed, all among residents of Chinatown. A short-term quarantine of Chinatown was instituted, fostered by fear and pervasive racial prejudice. Chinatown residents objected vehemently, instituting legal challenges, and the quarantine was lifted, ignoring Dr. Kinyoun's advice to the contrary. Health officials instituted house-to-house inspections of Chinatown in hopes of identifying further victims. However, fearing reprisals and other sanctions, the effort was hampered by the lack of cooperation by the Chinese, hiding bodies and locking doors.

Initially, with relatively few cases identified and fear of the adverse economic impact that news of a plague epidemic would have, "plague denial" was nearly universal among San Francisco's citizenry and local government officials. All were encouraged to ignore specious talk of plague, disparaged by government officials and many medical officers as "fake plague" news.

However, as case numbers increased within Chinatown and, ultimately, jumped the racial barrier to White citizens, denial was no longer an option. Then Surgeon General Walter Wyman replaced Dr. Kinyoun with the more amicable and practical-minded Dr. Rupert L. Blue (1868–1948) in hopes of eradicating the plague epidemic in a more timely and expeditious fashion. However, discouraged by persistent political in-fighting and lack of cooperation between state and local health authorities and the MHS, Dr. Blue quit his post in 2001, only to be called back into service in February 1903 as cases further multiplied.

Perhaps aware of Dr. Paul-Lois Simond's 1898 publication linking rats and fleas to the spread of plague [11], or arriving at the same conclusion based on his own observations [12], Dr. Blue declared war on Chinatown's rats. With new-found authority and cooperation with government and health officials, decrepit buildings were condemned and raised. Earthen basements were concreted, and streets and sidewalks paved. Houses were scoured with carbolic acid and lye and generous bounties paid for trapped rats.

---

[3]In 1894, two independent research physicians, Shibasaburo Kitasato [9] and Alexandre Yersin [10], had published manuscripts identifying the causative organism, now called *Yersinia pestis*.

Fig. 3.3 Autopsy/culture of rats during San Francisco's plague epidemic. (Picture Source: https://www.nature.com. The National Library of Medicine)

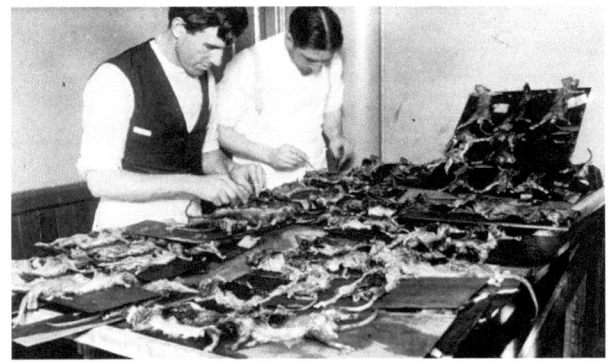

Blue's eradication campaign appeared to work. With cases on the wane and rat autopsies (Fig. 3.3) showing lack of bacterial contamination, Blue dismantled his team and left San Francisco in 1904. There had been a documented total of 121 cases in San Francisco and 5 outside the city limits, with a combined total of 122 deaths—the last recorded on February 29, 1904, in the town of Concord, California [8, 13].

Following San Francisco's 7.9 magnitude earthquake in 1906, approximately 80% of the city's infrastructure was destroyed, leaving 250,000 citizens homeless. Rats multiplied and massed over discarded garbage piles and open sewers and small outbreaks of plague reappeared. Blue was recalled to help contain the disease. Threatening to quarantine the entire city and prevent the US Navy fleet from docking, Blue was able to amass a small army of volunteer citizens to trap and kill rats, dispatching as many as 13,000 per week [12]. His containment tactics worked, and the city was declared plague-free in November 1908 [8, 14].

****

Two remarkable extensions of knowledge regarding plague and its epidemiology drew directly from Dr. Blue's and his colleague's research during and after the San Francisco epidemic [8]. First, while investigating a possible mode of transmission in a case occurring at considerable distance from San Francisco's city limits and its indigenous rat population, Blue captured and autopsied ground squirrels. To his surprise, they contained the plague bacillus!

It is now known that the plague bacterium (*Yersinia pestis*) is transmitted by fleas and cycles naturally through wild rodents including squirrels, prairie dogs, and wood rats in addition to urban rats, forming a persistent reservoir of infectious bacteria, maintained by parasitic fleas. An average of seven human plague cases have been reported per year in the USA in recent decades (Fig. 3.4), most in rural western states [15]. The last urban epidemic occurred in Los Angeles in 1924 through 1925.

Fig. 3.4 Reported cases of human plague: US 1970–2019. Each dot represents one case. (Picture Source: https://www.cdc.gov. CDC)

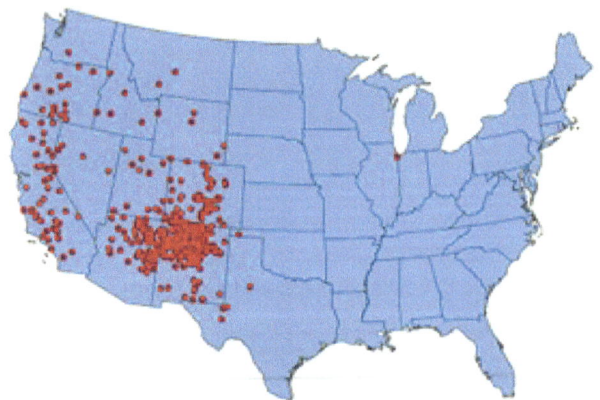

Second, colleagues of Blue initiated research on flea anatomy, elucidating their unique biting physiology but, most fortuitously, discovering that the predominate flea species in San Francisco was not the oriental rat flea, *Pulex cheopis* (*Xenopsylla cheopis*), but rather the northern European rat flea, *Ceratophyllus fasciatus* [8].

Subsequent anatomic research defined significant differences in the two species' gut physiology that made the San Francisco flea less efficient in introducing an inoculum of bacteria with each bite, providing a very plausible explanation as to why the San Francisco outbreak resulted in relatively few deaths compared to concurrent outbreaks in Asia [8].

In recognition of his contributions to public health, Dr. Blue was appointed to the position of Surgeon General by President Taft in 1812 and served a second term under President Wilson until 1920.

****

Today, plague is mostly a disease of historical interest, although pockets of infection remain around the world, particularly in central Asia where the disease is endemic. Antibiotic treatment with tetracyclines, chloramphenicol, or streptomycin is generally curative, although drug resistant strains have been identified in recent years [16].

Experimental vaccines against plague have been available since first introduced by Waldemar Haffkine (1860–1930) in 1896. Adverse side effects are common with existing vaccines and, according to the CDC, their efficacy has never been measured precisely, although field experience indicates their use reduces the incidence and severity of disease [16]. Most existing vaccines utilize killed or attenuated *Yersinia pestis*, with ongoing research to develop a safer and more effective vaccine for the commercial market [2].

According to the CDC, there is currently no need to vaccinate persons except for those with a uniquely high risk of exposure [16]. However, as *Yersinia pestis* is a category A pathogen, posing risk as an agent of bioterrorism, the need for public health preparedness is self-evident and vaccine research and development continues with considerable imperativeness [17].

Yellow Fever (*Bronze John, Yellow Jack*)

Yellow fever is an acute hemorrhagic disease, now known to be caused by an RNA arbovirus of the flavivirus genus [18], which is transmitted to humans through the bite of mosquitoes. Only female mosquitoes bite humans or other primates, a blood meal providing essential nutrients for egg production, most specifically iron [19]. Male mosquitoes feed on the nectar from flowers. The yellow fever virus is taken up by a female mosquito when it ingests the blood of an infected human or other primate and transfers the virus to another individual with a subsequent bite.

The mosquito-to-human transmission of the yellow fever virus varies somewhat depending on the environmental setting (Fig. 3.5). In the urban setting, the infecting

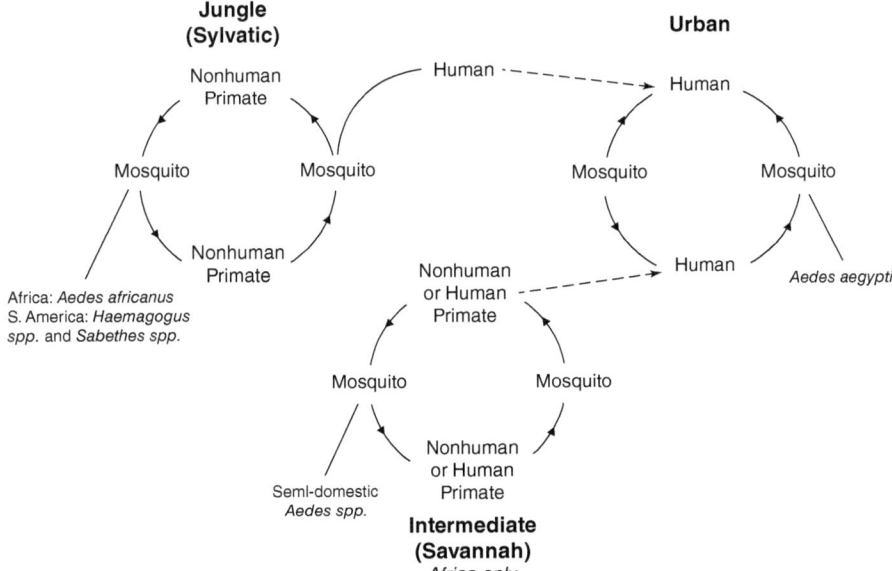

Fig. 3.5 Yellow fever transmission cycles. (Picture Source: https://www.cdc.gov. CDC)

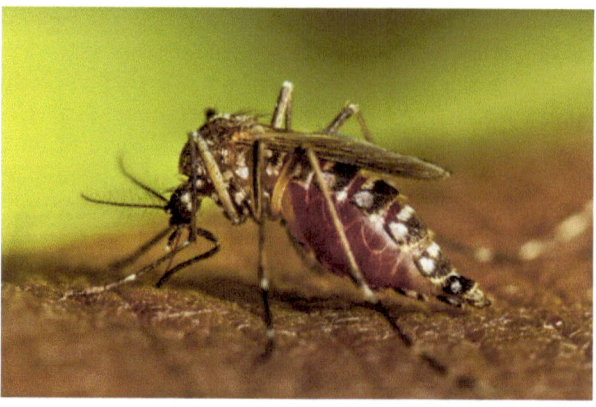

mosquito is the female *Aedes aegypti* which becomes disease transmissive about 2
weeks after feeding on an infected person with viremic symptoms, most notably
fever (Fig. 3.6). In the wild setting, sylvatic (jungle) yellow fever is transmitted by
Aedes, Haemagogus, and *Sabethes* forest canopy mosquitoes between non-human
primates, with occasional transmission to humans who happen to be residing or
traveling in an endemic area. In Africa, an intermediate (savannah) cycle also exists
in jungle border areas, with transmission modes from monkey to human and human
to human. Currently, the yellow fever virus is endemic in tropical areas of Africa
and Central and South America [18, 20].

The symptoms associated with yellow fever may be none, mild-to-moderate,
or severe, with fever, chills, headache, body ache, fatigue, restlessness, nausea,
and vomiting common in patients with mild-to-moderate cases. Recovery is typically within a week, with occasional protracted fatigue lasting several months. A
small portion of patients develop severe symptoms (sometimes preceded by a
brief remission), referred to as "malignant yellow fever." Symptoms include high
fever, slowed pulse (Faget sign), jaundiced (yellowed) eyes and skin, internal
bleeding with hematemesis, albuminuria, shock, and organ failure. Death in
severe cases is typically in the 30–60% range. Life-long immunity is usually
afforded to patients who have recovered from any form of symptomatic disease
[18, 20].

A diagnosis of yellow fever is typically made based on clinical presentation—
sudden fever, bradycardia, and jaundice—in a patient who has been in an endemic
area. As the symptom complex may be mimicked by other viral diseases (e.g., dengue hemorrhagic fever), viral culture, reverse transcription polymerase chain reaction (RT-PCR) or serological testing may be needed for an accurate diagnosis [21].
During recovery, pneumonia and other bacterial superinfections may occur.

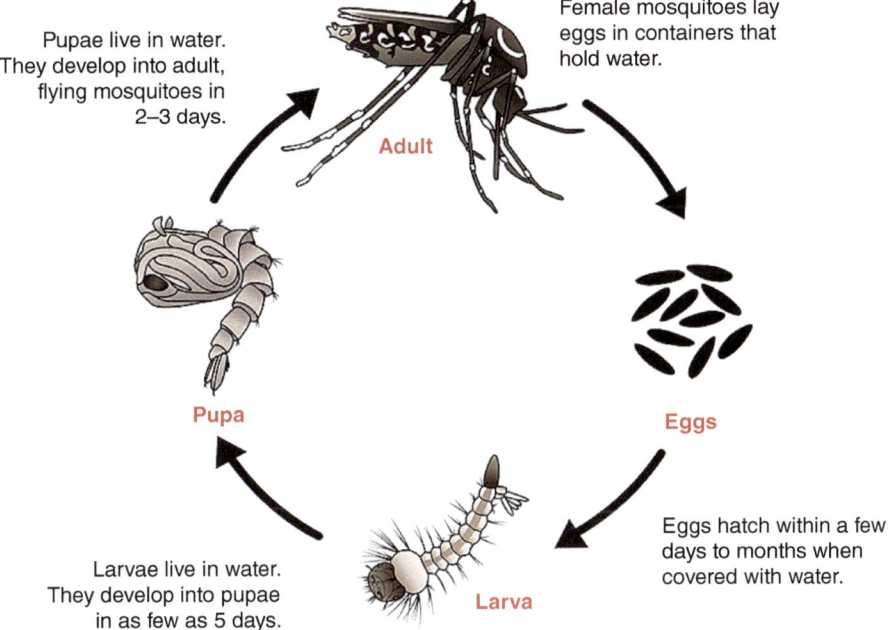

Pupae live in water.
They develop into adult,
flying mosquitoes in
2–3 days.

Adult

Female mosquitoes lay
eggs in containers that
hold water.

Pupa

Eggs

Larvae live in water.
They develop into pupae
in as few as 5 days.

Larva

Eggs hatch within a few
days to months when
covered with water.

Fig. 3.7 Life cycle of *Aedes aegypti* mosquito. (Picture Source: https://www.cdc.gov. CDC)

A safe and effective vaccine is available for yellow fever [20, 21]. Derived from an attenuated virus, a single dose affords life-long protection and is recommended for people aged 9 months or older who are living in or traveling to an endemic area. Significant side effects are reportedly rare [18]. There is no specific antiviral medication available for yellow fever, with treatment of symptomatic patients relegated to supportive care only.

Control of yellow fever in endemic areas is centered around four epidemiological principles: mass vaccination programs; vector control by eliminating mosquito breeding sites and the use of larvicides to disrupt the mosquito's life cycle (Fig. 3.7); surveillance monitoring of *Aedes* mosquito populations; and early containment of infection outbreaks [18]. In urban areas these initiatives by the World Health Organization (WHO) and its sister partners have had reasonable success [18]. The use of insecticides against adult mosquitoes has been less effective due to evolving vector resistance, safety concerns, and high cost. The elimination of jungle mosquitoes is not practical and considered untenable [18].

****

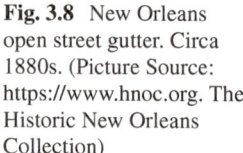

Fig. 3.8 New Orleans open street gutter. Circa 1880s. (Picture Source: https://www.hnoc.org. The Historic New Orleans Collection)

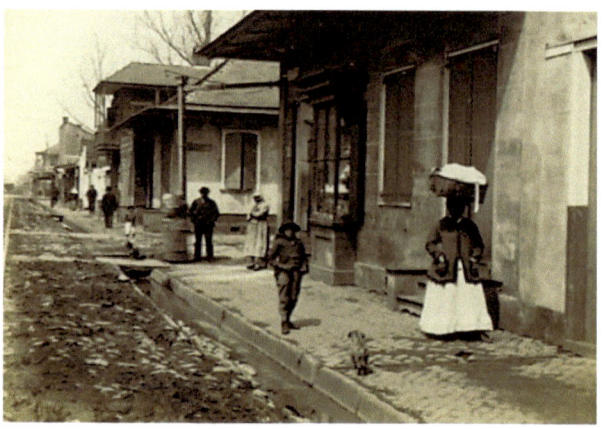

Brought to the western hemisphere from Africa during the slave trade era, yellow fever was one of the deadliest and most panic-provoking diseases to afflict the USA. From the first reported outbreak in 1648 in the Yucatan, Central America and the Caribbean suffered yellow fever epidemics for many years before the disease arrived in the British-American colonies in 1693 [22–24].

The *Aedes* mosquito vector was probably carried to coastal American cities via water barrels on trade ships transporting goods from the Caribbean, along with infected ship mates carrying the disease itself. Ships arriving from endemic areas were often quarantined offshore for 40 days or more to help contain the spread of disease. Those carrying crew or passengers with active infection were required to fly a yellow flag, giving the disease its common moniker, "yellow jack," by some accounts [22].

The initial 1693 outbreak in Boston was relatively contained, but the 1793 epidemic in Philadelphia was another matter.[4] With a 10% mortality and a large percentage of the population fleeing the town in fear of their lives, the capital city was economically and socially decimated [22, 23].

Another major outbreak occurred in Norfolk, Virginia, in 1855, but the worst outbreak of yellow fever in United States' history occurred in the Mississippi River Valley over the spring and summer of 1878 [22]. The area was surrounded by wetlands and city streets were fouled by stagnant water containing garbage and human and animal waste, providing ideal breeding grounds for mosquitoes, particularly in the warm and humid environment of the region (Fig. 3.8).

The 1878 epidemic started in New Orleans and spread up the Mississippi River to Memphis and inland, sickening a recorded 120,000 persons and causing between 13,000 and 20,000 deaths [23, 25]. With a mass exodus of persons fleeing

---

[4] The reader is referred to Ron Chernow's biography, *Alexander Hamilton* (Penguin Books, 2005) and/or the historical novel *My Dear Hamilton: A Novel of Eliza Schuyler Hamilton* by Stephanie Dray and Laura Kamoie (William Morrow/HarperCollins Publishers, New York, NY, 2018) for insight into the social and economic impact of the 1793 Philadelphia epidemic.

contagion, the economy of the region suffered enormously. Observed at the time was the fact that recent White immigrants to the area were the most susceptible, while local White and Black residents enjoyed relative disease resistance, probably proportional to the level of naturally acquired immunity in the different populations [22, 26].

While the institution of strict quarantine and isolation measures to limit importation and spread of yellow fever, coupled with massive public works projects to improve sanitation and city cleanliness, were helpful in breaking endemic cycles of disease in urban areas in the USA, it was a decades-long endeavor to discover the root cause of yellow fever.

Until late in the nineteenth century the principal theory explaining the origin and spread of disease was atmospheric miasma. Little appreciated was the fact that construction of underground sewer systems, installation of municipal water supplies, drainage of swamps, institution of city-wide trash and garbage collection, and other large-scale public works projects to rid cities of foul smells, also eliminated breeding grounds for mosquitoes and diminished fecal contamination of drinking water. A lessened incidence of yellow fever, cholera, and other diseases following completion of these types of urban renewal endeavors only served to reinforce the miasma theory. Germ theory, as introduced by the ground-breaking work of Louis Pasteur (1822–1895) and Joseph Lister (1827–1912), and solidified by the subsequent identification of several disease-causing bacteria by Robert Koch (1843–1910), was late in acceptance in the USA, as previously discussed.

The pioneering work of Cuban physician Carlos Juan Finlay (1833–1915) in the 1880s and 1890s laid the groundwork for U.S. Army scientists working under direction of Dr. Walter Reed (1851–1902) (Fig. 3.9) to confirm Finlay's unproved

Fig. 3.9 Major Walter Reed. Unidentified photographer. (Picture Source: https://commons. wikimedia.org)

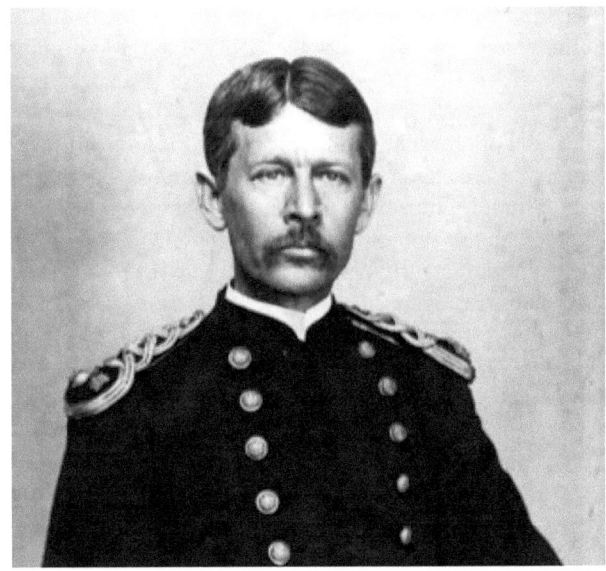

contention that the *Aedes aegypti* (formerly called *Culex fasciatus)* mosquito was the vector responsible for spreading yellow fever [22–24]. The imperative for Reed's work was the unprecedented death rate of U.S. soldiers from yellow fever during the Spanish American war in Cuba.

Using human volunteers in his research, Dr. Reed was able to establish the following (paraphrased) conclusions regarding the epidemiology of yellow fever, which he presented to the Pan-American Medical Congress in Havana, Cuba, on February 6, 1901 [22, 23]:

- The mosquito *Aedes aegypti* serves as an intermediate host for the "parasite" [causative agent] of yellow fever.
- Yellow fever is transferred from an infected person to a non-immune person by the bite of an *Aedes aegypti* mosquito.
- An extrinsic incubation period of about 12 days in the mosquito is needed for infective transmission.
- Yellow fever can be transferred to a non-immune person by subcutaneous injection of blood from an infected person if the blood is harvested during the first 2 days of illness.
- The incubation period in humans ranges from 2 to 6 days.
- Yellow fever is not transferred by fomites [contaminated clothes or bedding] or spread within a house, unless harboring infected mosquitoes.
- The spread of yellow fever can be best controlled by the destruction of mosquitoes and the protection of infected persons from subsequent bites of propagating mosquito vectors.

Reed's conclusions led General William C. Gorgas (1854–1929) to institute massive campaigns against the urban mosquito vector, eliminating yellow fever in Havana in 1902 and in the Panama Canal zone 4 years later—defeating the disease that had stymied the French effort to build the canal. Similar eradication campaigns eliminated yellow fever in the USA, with the last major outbreak in New Orleans in 1905 [22–24].

The Rockefeller Foundation formed the Yellow Fever Commission in 1918, with the goal of eliminating the *Aedes aegypti* mosquito, worldwide. Urban campaigns in endemic areas were reasonably successful, but the discovery of the zoonotic sylvatic (jungle) mosquito species made the goal of global elimination of yellow fever unrealistic, as noted previously.

Although clearly defining the mode of propagation, Reed was unable to identify the causative agent of yellow fever. It took scientists another 25 years to determine that the "filterable agent" described by Reed was a virus, first identified by Adrian Stokes (1887–1927) in 1927. Max Theiler (1899–1972) of the Rockefeller Foundation received the Nobel Prize in Physiology or Medicine in 1951 for his development of an effective vaccine against yellow fever in the 1930s, providing the principal tool for disease control today.

In an effort to control the spread of yellow fever and other viruses, including dengue, Zika, and chikungunya, which are also carried and transmitted by the female *Aedes aegypti* mosquito, experimentation is currently underway using genetically modified (GM) mosquitoes [27]. These mosquitoes are laboratory bred and contain a gene that prevents female mosquito offspring from surviving into adulthood, as well as a fluorescent marker gene to help identify modified mosquitoes in the wild. When released into areas of endemic disease, it is hoped that the modified mosquitoes will interbreed with native mosquitoes, ultimately decreasing the population of infecting mosquitoes. Produced by the biotechnology firm Oxitec, experimental releases of GM mosquitoes are currently being carried out in the USA under preview of the EPA [28].

Typhus (*Ship Fever, Jail Fever*)

Although they have similar names and similar symptoms, typhus is a very different disease from typhoid fever. The diseases are caused by different bacteria and have entirely different modes of transmission. Typhoid fever is spread by fecal contamination of food and water. Typhus is a vector-borne disease.

****

Three varieties of typhus are commonly recognized [29–32]:

1. Epidemic typhus is caused by the bacterium *Rickettsia prowazekii* and is principally spread from person-to-person by infected human body lice (Fig. 3.10)—more specifically, when bacteria laden louse feces are scratched into bite wounds or rubbed into mucous membranes of the eyes or mouth. Inhalation of dried louse feces is also a mechanism of infection as is exposure to flying squirrels or their nests, the bacteria speculatively transferred via a secondary louse or flea bite.

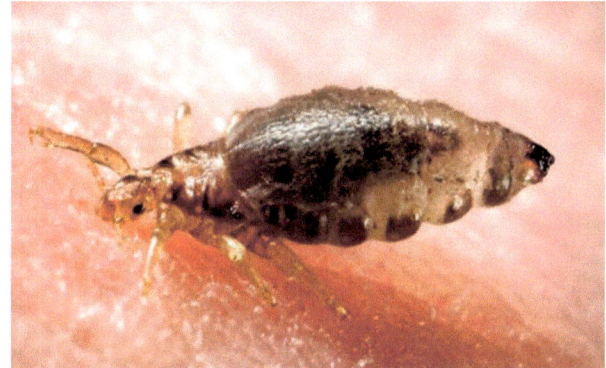

Fig. 3.10 The human body louse *Pediculus humanus corporis*. (Picture Source: https://www.cdc.gov. CDC)

2. Scrub (bush) typhus is caused by the bacterium *Orientia tsutsugamushi* and is spread to people by the bite of infected chiggers (larval mites).
3. Flea-borne (murine) typhus is caused by the bacterium *Rickettsia typhus*, transmitted to humans by the bite of a flea carrying typhus bacteria derived from infected rats, cats or opossums. As with epidemic typhus, the flea's feces (flea dirt) carry the bacteria which are typically transferred into the bite wound by scratching. Rubbing the eye with a contaminated finger or inhalation of flea dirt are other possible modes of infection.

The clinical signs and symptoms are similar for the three varieties of typhus including: high fever, headache, rapid breathing, body aches and muscle pain, nausea, vomiting, confusion, and rash (Fig. 3.11). An eschar (scab) may occur at the site of a chigger bite. Symptoms typically occur 10 days to 2 weeks after the vector bite. Persons with severe illness may develop organ failure and internal hemorrhage, which can be fatal if untreated.

Recurrent symptoms (generally milder) of epidemic typhus—known as Brill-Zinger disease—can occur many years after complete recovery from the initial infection, most commonly in the elderly or if the immune system is otherwise compromised.

All three types of typhus are treated with supportive care and antibiotics. The current antibiotic of choice is doxycycline, with prompt recovery likely if started

Fig. 3.11 Skin rash of murine typhus. (Picture Source: https://www.ncbi. nlm.nih.gov. West J Emerg Med: 10(3), 2009/Creative Commons Article)

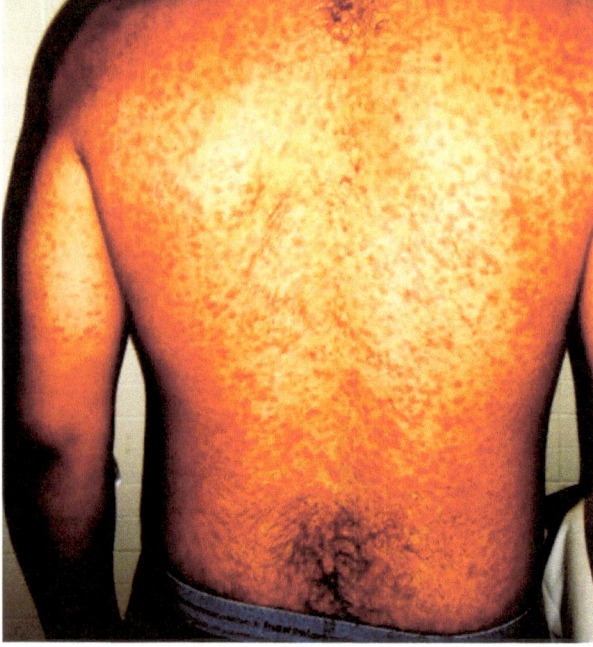

soon after symptoms begin [29, 30]. Diagnosis is based on clinical findings coupled with epidemiological evidence of body louse exposure, most commonly where people are clustered together under unhygienic conditions.

Early diagnostic tests are not available, but a typhus infection can be confirmed by bacterial culture, serological tests to detect IgG or IgM antibodies or polymerase chain reaction (PCR) assays of blood, plasma or tissue [29, 30]. There are no vaccines available against typhus. As such, preventive measures to avoid body louse infestations, including frequent bathing, hot water washing of clothes and bedding, and spraying clothing and bedding with 0.5% permethrin, are recommended in conditions of unhygienic overcrowding [29, 30].

****

Although epidemic typhus is currently a rare disease, it was responsible for millions of deaths in previous centuries, particularly where people were residing in crowded and unhygienic conditions. Human lice thrive on unwashed clothing, bedding, and hair—a nearly universal state of being well into the nineteenth century, both here and abroad. Endemic among steerage class emigrants and within crowded jails, where body lice could easily jump from one individual to the next, the disease was known as "ship fever" or "jail fever," among many other monikers appropriate to other crowded living conditions.

American physician William Wood Gerhard (1809–1872) was the first to accurately distinguish typhus from typhoid fever based on comparative postmortem examination of typhus patients afflicted in the 1836 outbreak in Philadelphia's Blockley Almshouse (later named Philadelphia General Hospital). He observed that typhus patients did not have the "morbid" changes in the bowel (swelling, hemorrhage, necrosis, and perforation) typically present in typhoid patients [33, 34]. Unfortunately, he was unable to provide any life-saving insight into the etiology or mode of contagion of either disease, other than the observation that those afflicted lived in close proximity to one another.

Unlike European countries, the USA has been relatively spared the scourge of epidemic typhus, perhaps due to an unrecognized anatomical difference in the North American louse population compared to that of the Europe variety, making contagion less efficient [35]. Typhus outbreaks were rare among Civil War soldiers or in prisoner-of-war camps, despite crowded and unhygienic living conditions [35]. Similarly, typhus outbreaks on the Western Front during WWI were also uncommon, notwithstanding soldiers being constantly tormented by body lice, commonly referred to as "cooties."[5]

---

[5] Of interest, trench fever is another disease transmitted by the body louse. First described during WW I, trench fever ravaged combat troops during the Great War and is caused by the bacterium

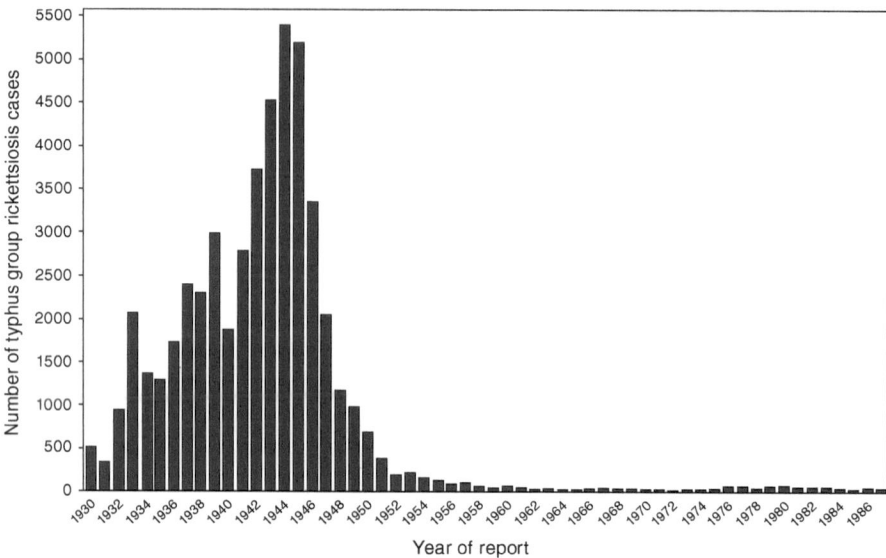

Fig. 3.12 Flea-borne typhus cases in the USA by Year (1930–1986). (Picture Source: https://www.cdc.gov. CDC)

In contrast, the Russian soldiers on the Eastern Front were decimated by typhus—causing an estimated 30,000,000 cases and 3,000,000 deaths—suggesting that the typhus bacterium was not present within the Western European trenches [36, 37]. Speculatively, if typhus bacteria had spread to France, WWI might have had an entirely different outcome [37].

According to the CDC, several thousand cases of flea-borne typhus were reported each year in the USA during the 1930s and 1940s [38]. By 1958 less than 100 cases were reported each year and only a few cases still occur on a yearly basis (Fig. 3.12), primarily in California, Hawaii and Texas [38].

Malaria (*Swamp Fever, Ague, Congestive Fever*)

An ancient disease [39] characterized by relapsing fevers and death; malaria remains one of the most devastating afflictions in the modern world. Its Roman name, *mal'aria* ("bad air") derives from its long association with foul stagnant water, and the pervasive belief at the time that malodorous air (miasmas) was the source of disease [40].

Bartonella quintana [36].

Malaria is caused by the protozoa parasite *Plasmodium*, which is transmitted to humans through the bite of an infected female *Anopheles* mosquito. First identified by French physician Charles L. A. Laveran (1845–1922) in 1880, five related subtypes of *Plasmodium* are now known to be responsible for malarial infections [39, 40]:

- *P. falciparum*
- *P. vivax*
- *P. ovale*
- *P. malaria*
- *P. knowlesi*

Of the five types, *P. vivax* and *P. falciparum* are the most common, and *P. falciparum* is most likely to cause severe malaria and death, if left untreated [41, 42].

Although no longer a significant threat in the USA and most of Europe, nearly half or the world's population remains at risk of malaria, with infants, children under 5 years of age, pregnant women, and persons with HIV/AIDS or low acquired immunity at greatest risk for severe disease, according to the WHO [42]. In 2021, the WHO estimates that there were 247 million cases of malaria worldwide with an estimated 619,000 deaths, with the WHO Africa Region experiencing 95% of cases and 96% of deaths [43].

Symptoms of malaria infection may vary from mild to severe and may cause death. Commonly, people experience fever, chills, sweats, headaches, nausea and vomiting, body aches, and general malaise—classically in repetitive cycles of varying duration and interval (*ague*) depending on the infecting *Plasmodium* species. Signs of infection include an elevated temperature, perspiration, weakness, enlarged spleen and/or liver, jaundice, and tachypnea (a rapid respiratory rate) [42].

Severe malaria may involve the brain (cerebral malaria) or kidneys and may invoke coagulopathies, respiratory distress, severe anemia, metabolic acidosis, cardiovascular collapse, and death. After recovery, patients with *P. vivax* and *P. ovale* infections may experience symptomatic relapses months or years later due to reactivation of dormant liver-stage parasites (hypnozoites) [42].

Surgeon-Major Ronald Ross (1857–1932) of the British Indian Medical Service is credited with identifying the *Anopheles* mosquito as the transmitting vector for malaria in 1897, for which he received the Nobel Prize in 1902 [40]. The subsequent delineation of the life cycle of the *Plasmodium* parasite within the infecting mosquito and human host is attributable to multiple contributing scientists over the years [40, 44].

Simplistically, an immature form of the malaria parasite (sporozoite) is injected into the human bloodstream during a blood meal bite by the female *Anopheles* mosquito. The sporozoites are carried to the liver where they asexually reproduce and mature into forms known as schizonts. Schizonts release merozoites which break out of the liver and invade red blood cells where they grow and divide and, ultimately, rupture the cell. In the process, toxic substances are released, causing the characteristic malaria symptoms. In a parallel pathway, sexually formed gameto-cytes produced in the human host are transferred to an uninfected mosquito in a subsequent bite, perpetuating the vector/host cycle of disease transmission (Fig. 3.13) [42].

The diagnosis of malaria is based on the patient's clinical presentation, coupled with microscopic examination of blood smears to identify the *Plasmodium* parasite. Several antigen-based rapid diagnostic tests (RDTs) are available and are helpful when skilled microscopists are not readily accessible. Polymerase chain reaction tests for parasite nucleic acid detection are also available and are particularly help-ful in the identification of the infecting species but may not be readily obtainable for rapid confirmation of infection in many areas of the world [42].

The oldest pharmaceutical compound for the treatment of malaria is quinine. Still in use today, quinine was originally derived from the bark of the Peruvian cin-chona tree. Lack of availability, developing parasite drug resistance and unpleasant side effects lead to the search for alternative drugs. The decimation of Allied and Central Powers/Axis troops during WWI and WWII from malaria infections fos-tered intense research efforts leading to the sequential development of quinacrine (Atabrine) and chloroquine, followed by sulfadoxine-pyrimethamine.

Nasty side effects and the appearance of chloroquine-resistant falciparum malaria spurred the development of mefloquine through a collaborative effort of the U.S. Army Medical Research and Development Command, the WHO, and

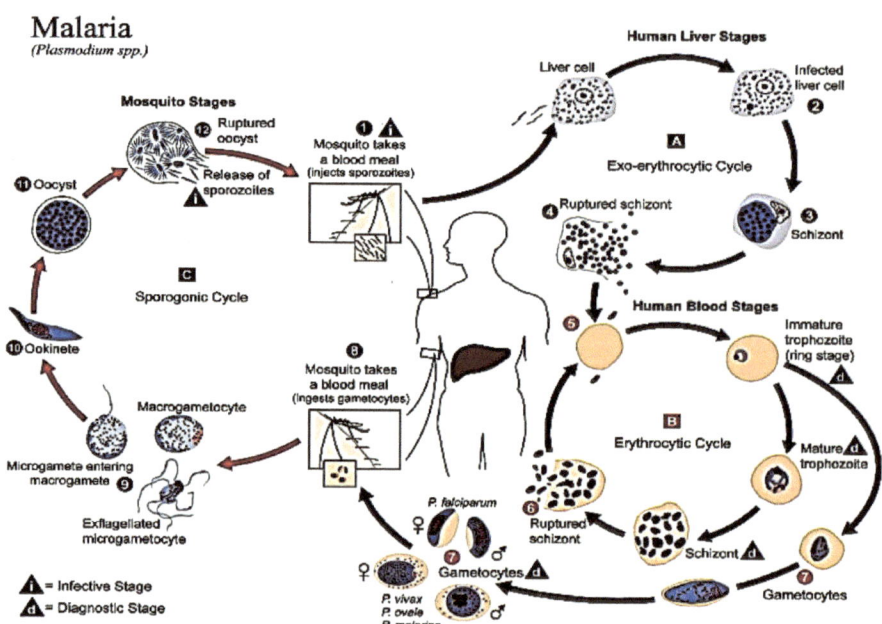

Fig. 3.13 Malaria *Plasmodium* parasite lifecycle. (Picture Source: https://www.cdc.gov/malaria/about/biology. CDC)

Hoffman-La Roche, Inc. Persistent drug resistant strains prompted further research by Chinese scientists, leading to the development of artemisinin in the 1970s, originally isolated from the Artemisia annua (sweet worm) plant [40, 45].

As treatment regimens depend on the infecting species of *Plasmodium* and its known or expected drug susceptibility, as well as the clinical status of the patient and the patient's history of previous treatment or current use of malarial prophylactic drugs, the selection of antimalarial drugs in isolation or combination remains in the province of an infectious disease expert [42]. That said, the WHO recommends an artemisinin-based combination therapy in most cases, particularly for *P. Falciparum,* to ensure a rapid and complete elimination of the malaria parasite [43].

A vaccine against malaria is currently available, produced by GSK pharmaceutical company. Known as RTS,S (marketed as Mosquirix) and endorsed by the WHO in 2021 [43], the vaccine was many years in development and is the first vaccine available against malaria or any other parasitic disease. A *Plasmodium* circumsporozoite protein antigen vaccine, RTS,S was shown to have an efficacy of around 50% in children 5–17 months of age in phase 3 trials and is anticipated to save tens of thousands of lives each year if widely administered—most notably by decreasing the incidence of severe malaria caused by the *P. falciparum* species [46–48].

Persons repeatedly exposed to malaria parasites appear to develop a degree of natural immunity, most specifically against severe disease caused by *P. falciparum* [49]. Poorly understood, acquired immunity is relatively short lived if a person is removed from repetitive exposures. Without a naturally acquired or vaccine induced immunity, recurrent malaria infections can occur with severe anemia, splenomegaly or rupture, and nephrotic syndrome being recognized complications associated with different species of *Plasmodium* [42].

Of evolutionary interest, persons with *sickle cell trait* (SCT)—having inherited an abnormal hemoglobin "S" gene from one parent and a normal hemoglobin "A" gene from the other parent—suffer few complications of sickle cell disease but are particularly resistant to severe malarial episodes, providing a selective survival advantage in areas (such as southern Africa) where malaria is endemic [40, 50].

****

Endemic and epidemic malaria plagued the USA until the early twentieth century. It weakened troop strength during the American Revolution and Civil War, migrated west with the California Gold Rush and decimated Native American peoples. Citizens residing in southern states and territories were victimized by the disease throughout American history until its pervasive threat was eliminated in the early 1950s [40, 51].

Following identification of the *Plasmodium* parasite (1880) and the mosquito vector (1897), malaria eradication efforts in America paralleled those targeting yellow fever, namely elimination of mosquito breeding habitats. Following the Spanish American War and during construction of the Panama Canal, huge strides were made in mosquito control in Cuba and in the canal zone, as well as southern states, by draining swamps, filling marshes, and eliminating stagnant pools of fresh water. Sanitary sewer systems were installed in many cities, eliminating open sewage contaminating streets and creeks which provided ideal breeding grounds for the domestic *Anopheles* mosquito [51, 52].

An amalgamation of malaria control with economic development occurred in the USA with the formation of the Tennessee Valley Authority (TVA) in 1933. Along with the construction of hydroelectric dams, mosquito breeding sites were eliminated by raising water levels and insecticide application, virtually eliminating the disease in the Tennessee River valley from a pre-construction prevalence affecting nearly 30% of the area's population [52].

As malaria came under control in the States, new concerns arose during World War II as soldiers succumbed in droves to malaria in the Pacific Theater. Affecting 60–65% of Pacific Theater troops during the course of the war, malaria markedly impacted combat preparedness [53]. Combating the disease focused on administering prophylactic antimalarial drugs (principally Atabrine due to the lack of quinine availability) and spraying mosquito breeding sites with oil and the DDT insecticide. Educational campaigns were instituted to exhort GIs to wear protective clothing, use mosquito nets, apply insect repellent (DEET), forgo evening swimming and take the prescribed antimalarial medication despite its nasty side effects. Multiple propaganda posters (Fig. 3.14) were produced (many incorporating scantily clad women) encouraging compliance with these antimalaria recommendations, the net effect being an estimated 70% reduction in malaria rates [53].

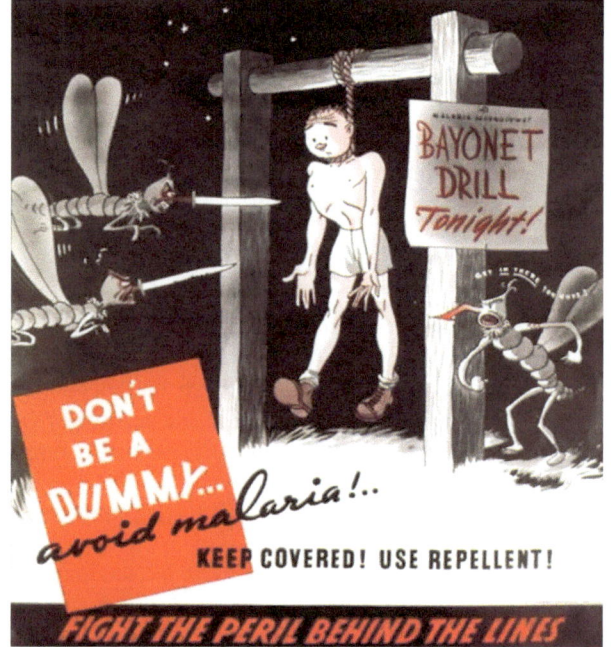

Fig. 3.14 WWII propaganda poster encouraging malaria preventive measures. (Picture Source: https://www.motherjones.com. National Library of Medicine)

Fig. 3.15 Insecticide
spraying in Savannah,
Georgia,
by the MCWA. (Picture
Source: https://www.cdc.
gov. CDC: Public Health
Image Library)

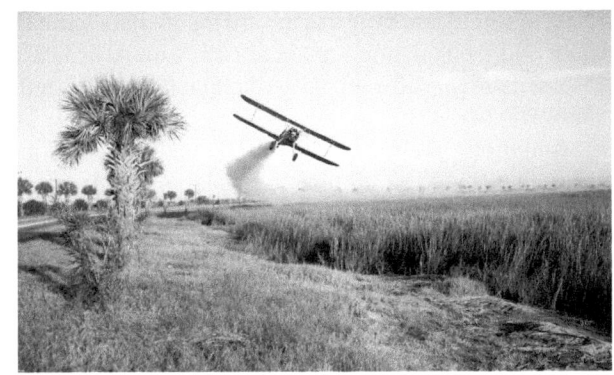

Reintroduction of malaria to a vulnerable civilian population by returning soldiers carrying the parasite was a major concern during the war years, prompting the formation of the Malaria Control in War Areas (MCWA) initiative in 1942. The MCWA's mission was to treat infected soldiers with antimalarials and contain the possible spread of malaria and other vector-borne diseases around military bases through the use of netting, household insecticide (DDT) fumigation, and elimination of mosquito breeding sites through drainage and insecticide spraying (Fig. 3.15) [51, 52].

The CDC (originally known as the Communicable Disease Center) stemmed from the MCWA initiative and began its inception in 1946 with one of its original missions to eradicate malaria as a public health threat. In a combined effort between the CDC and the National Malaria Eradication Program, malaria was eliminated in the USA by 1951. At that point, the CDC switched its malaria emphasis from disease elimination to a focus on prevention and surveillance within the States and technical support to economically undeveloped areas of the world, in a cooperative effort to eliminate malaria worldwide [52].

Currently, around 2000 cases of malaria are diagnosed in the USA each year, the vast majority being in persons returning from countries where malaria remains endemic, principally from sub-Saharan Africa and South Asia [42]. However, locally acquired malaria remains a persistent threat, as evidenced by an outbreak of eight cases in Palm Beach County, Florida, in 2003, and the recent identification (July 2023) of six locally acquired cases of *Plasmodium vivax* malaria in Sarasota County, Florida, and one in Cameron County, Texas [54].

Treatment and isolation of infected persons, coupled with truck and aerial insecticide spraying of area mosquito breeding sites remains the principal method of containment in these small outbreaks [54]. However, in a world of rapid global travel and the omnipresent *Anopheles* mosquito vector, the threat of recurring malaria outbreaks remains of concern [55].

****

Despite significant progress toward the global elimination of malaria, nearly half of the world's population remain at risk, with Africa carrying a lopsided share of the disease burden, suffering 95% of all malaria cases and 96% of deaths, according to the WHO [41, 43].

Ambitious goals set by the WHO include a 90% reduction of malaria case and death rates by 2030, eliminating malaria in at least 35 countries by 2030, and preventing malaria resurgence in all countries that are currently malaria free [43]. Preventive measures center on three fundamental strategies [43]:

• Vector Control
• Preventive Chemotherapies
• Vaccination

Vector control plays an obvious and vital role in preventing malaria transmission by *Anopheles* mosquitoes. Methods in use by the WHO and other global and regional agencies include indoor residual spraying (IRS) with insecticide, use of insecticide-treated nets (ITNs), larviciding to decrease mosquito populations, and environmental management to remove mosquito breeding sites. Widespread insecticide spraying is no longer embraced for fear of fomenting the emergence of resistant mosquito stains and the resultant loss of an effective tool in the containment of localized outbreaks [43, 54].

Preventive chemotherapy with therapeutic medications is used to prevent (or treat) outbreaks of malaria in vulnerable populations [43, 54]. Ideally, a full course of antimalarial medication will cure any existing infections and prevent new infections during the post-treatment prophylaxis period. Referred to as "mass" drug administration (MDA), "targeted" drug administration (TDA), or "reactive" drug administration (RDA) depending on the circumstantial objectives [55–57], eliminating the parasite in the targeted host population will, theoretically, break the vector/host transmission cycle and prevent further outbreaks.

Vaccination with RTS,S/AS01 malaria vaccine has been shown to reduce malaria and deadly severe malaria in children living in regions with a high incidence of *P. falciparum* transmission and is projected to save thousands of lives each year if widely administered [43, 47].

Dengue (*Breakbone Fever, Seven-day Fever*)

Currently, dengue is an uncommon infection within the continental United States but remains a significant threat to travelers visiting the Caribbean, Puerto Rico, Central or South America, or almost any other tropical or subtropical area of the world, where the disease is rampant. Dengue is caused by four virus serotypes (DENV-1 to DENV-4) and is transmitted from person-to-person by *Aedes aegypti* or

Ae. Albopictus mosquitoes, which are the same mosquito varieties that transmit yellow fever, Zika, chikungunya, and other viruses [58, 59].

Dengue is the leading cause of arthropod-borne disease in the world with an estimated 400 million infections, 100 million symptomatic cases and 40,000 deaths per year, according to the CDC [59]. Most people with dengue infections remain asymptomatic but around one in four get sick. The typical febrile course usually lasts around a week and is often accompanied by muscle, joint, and bone pain, accounting for the disease's common appellations. Other symptoms often include eye pain, headache, nausea and vomiting, and rash (Fig. 3.16) [59, 60].

Severe dengue (*dengue hemorrhagic shock*) affects around 1 in 20 persons who are sick with the infection [59]. With a typical onset a day or two after subsidence of the initial infection's accompanying fever, severe dengue can develop within a few hours and result in shock, internal bleeding, and death. Abdominal pain, bleeding from the gums or nose, bloody vomitus, stool or urine, difficulty breathing, fatigue, and irritability are all warning signs and symptoms of an impending life-threatening crisis requiring immediate medical attention [59, 60].

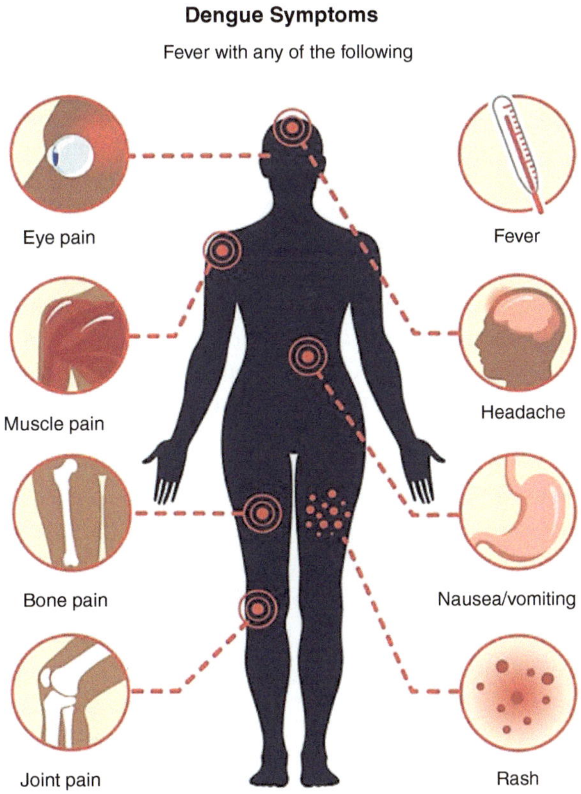

Fig. 3.16 Dengue symptoms. (Picture Source: https://www.cdc.gov/dengue. CDC)

Dengue Symptoms

Fever with any of the following

Eye pain

Muscle pain

Bone pain

Joint pain

Fever

Headache

Nausea/vomiting

Rash

A pregnant woman can pass the infecting virus to her fetus during pregnancy or during the birthing process, with a higher incidence of premature birth, low birth weight, and fetal distress. Spread through blood transfusions, organ transplants or needle sticks is also possible [59, 60].

****

There is no specific treatment for dengue other than symptomatic care. A previous infection affords long-term immunity to the specific infecting virus type but not the remaining three varieties [60]. Of critical importance, persons previously infected with dengue are more likely to develop severe dengue with a new infection, as are infants and pregnant women [59].

The diagnosis of dengue is based on exposure history and clinical presentation, coupled with molecular tests (*Nucleic Acid Amplification Test*: NAAT), antigen detection tests, and serological (IgM) tests for dengue viruses [59].

A dengue quadrivalent vaccine is available from Sanofi Pasteur, Inc. (*Dengvaxia*), which is currently approved in the USA only for people ages 9–16 who have had dengue fever at least once and are seropositive (laboratory confirmed infection) and live in an endemic area, including American Samoa, Guam, Puerto Rico, and the U.S. Virgin Islands [61, 62]. Persons with no prior history of infection (seronegative) appear to be at greater risk of developing severe dengue if they are infected after receiving the vaccine and are not approved for vaccination at this time. Prophylactic travel vaccination is not currently recommended for U.S. citizens, even to endemic areas [61, 63].

Currently, infection prophylaxis is centered around preventing mosquito bites. Avoidance measures include staying in air-conditioned or well screened housing, wearing protective clothing (long sleeved shirts, long pants, sock, and shoes), using mosquito repellant (permethrin impregnated clothing and DEET skin repellant) and eliminating standing water breeding sites in the immediate vicinity of residential housing [59, 60]. Widespread insecticide spraying (DDT) and large-scale drainage of swamps and wetlands was very effective in decreasing the domestic mosquito population and the yellow fever threat in Cuba, Central America, and the southern United States in the years following the Spanish American War. However, as noted in the Yellow Fever and other vector-borne disease sections, these types of control measures are no longer widely embraced because of their cost, negative environmental impact and the emergence of insecticide resistant mosquitoes. As a result, there has been a huge resurgence of the *Ae. Aegypti* population and an unprecedented increase in dengue cases in the Americas in recent years [63].

****

Outbreaks of dengue were common in the USA and its territories in the eighteenth and nineteenth century. A 1780 outbreak in Philadelphia is clearly described by Dr. Walter Reed, for example. In 1850 several cities in the southern states reported dengue-like illnesses, as did many others in subsequent years [64].

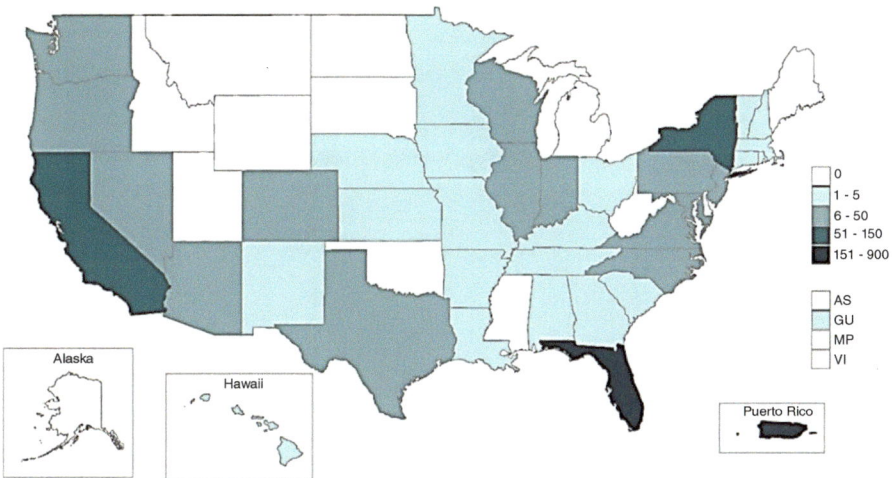

Fig. 3.17 States and territories reporting dengue cases, 2022. (Picture Source: https://www.cdc.gov/dengue/statistics-maps/2022. CDC)

The unprecedented 1901 initiative to eliminate the *Ae. Aegypti* mosquito in Havana, Cuba, undertaken by William Gorgas in the wake of Dr. Walter Reed's landmark study linking the mosquito vector to the spread of yellow fever, was hugely successful. It was followed by equally successful campaigns in the Panama Canal Zone and in southern cities in the USA, all of which resulted in a dramatic decrease in dengue incidence and other mosquito-borne diseases in the control areas.

That said, the *Aedes* mosquito was not entirely eliminated in these initiatives and, as noted above, there has been a huge resurgence of dengue cases in Cuba and other Caribbean islands, Central America, South America and throughout the tropical and subtropical world where mosquitoes thrive and human populations have expanded[6] [64].

Currently, most cases within the continental U.S. are imported with travelers returning from endemic areas, but locally transmitted cases are occurring with increasing frequency, as well. Below is a CDC map (Fig. 3.17) depicting the reported incidences of dengue in America in 2022 [65]. Florida, for example, had 750 travel-associated cases and 57 locally transmitted cases. Puerto Rico had 6 travel-associated cases and 820 locally transmitted cases. Overall, there were 1188 reported cases in U.S. states and 828 cases in U.S. territories in 2022 [65].

---

[6] *The Washington Post* (author: Jintak Han) reported on June 17, 2023, that Peru had extended a health emergency declaration in 18 of its 24 regions following more than 140,000 recorded cases of Dengue and at least 200 deaths. The epidemic represents the largest outbreak of Dengue in the county's history.

Fig. 3.18 Schematic
drawing of the bullet-
shaped rabies virus.
(Picture Source: https://
www.cdc.gov/rabies. CDC)

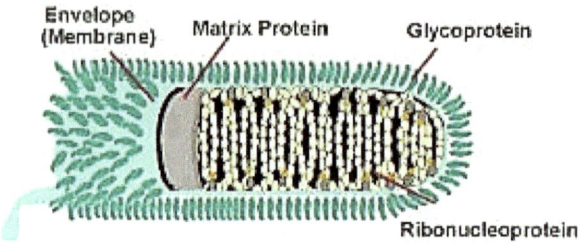

Rabies

Rabies is a vaccine-preventable zoonotic disease caused by bullet-shaped RNA viruses (principally *Rabies lyssavirus*) (Fig. 3.18), most often transmitted to people through the open-wound bite of a rabid animal containing virus-laden saliva [66, 67]. It is one of the deadliest and most horrific diseases to afflict humans, with a mortality close to 100% in untreated cases. An ancient affliction, the aggressive behavior and foaming mouths of rabid dogs, bats, and other mammals biting human beings is the likely basis for the fanciful images of werewolves, vampires, and other diabolical creatures conjured up in the minds of men [68].

The rabies virus infects the central nervous system of humans and other mammals, ultimately causing disease in the brain and death. After wound (or contaminated scratch) inoculation, the virus travels through the peripheral nerves to the brain. The transit time is variable but is usually 1–3 months [69, 70]. Upon reaching the brain, the viruses rapidly multiply and pass to the salivary glands. With brain involvement, unmistakable signs of rabies become apparent, ultimately leading to coma and death.

Rabies symptoms and signs depend on the stage of the infection. In humans, five stages are generally recognized: incubation, prodrome, acute neurological, coma, and death. Virus inoculation occurs at the time of the animal bite, when virus-laden saliva enters the wound and viruses begin to multiply. This incubation stage is asymptomatic with respect to the rabies infection.

When the virus enters the peripheral nervous system (prodromal stage), flu-like symptoms are common. Unusual tingling or burning sensations at the wound site may occur. Acute neurological symptoms follow when the virus enters the central nervous system and may fall into two different patterns: "furious rabies symptoms" (encephalitic) or "paralytic rabies symptoms." Furious symptoms generally include agitation and aggression, restlessness, seizures, fever, tachycardia, excessive salivation, facial muscle paralysis, fear of water (hydrophobia) and air (aerophobia), and delirium, among others. Paralytic symptoms occur in about 20% of patients and include fever, headache, stiff neck, weakness, paralysis, and coma. Death rapidly ensues in virtually all cases [70–72].

Although any mammal can get rabies, the vast majority of rabies cases reported to the CDC each year occur in wild animals such as bats, raccoons, skunks, and foxes. Worldwide, domestic dogs are the overwhelming source of human rabies, accounting for up to 99% of cases [71]. With nearly universal rabies vaccination of pet dogs, bats (Fig. 3.19) have supplanted canines as the most common cause of human infections within the USA [70].

The CDC recommends strict avoidance of wild animals, particularly bats, as a bat bite or scratch may seem innocuous and is easily overlooked or difficult to detect. Bats should never be kept as pets and if found within a house should be safely captured (if possible) and tested for rabies [70].

In addition to bats, terrestrial mammals such as raccoons, skunks, and foxes are important reservoirs of rabies, with their specific prevalence found in different areas of the country (Fig. 3.20). Vaccinated dogs and cats rarely become infected with rabies [70].

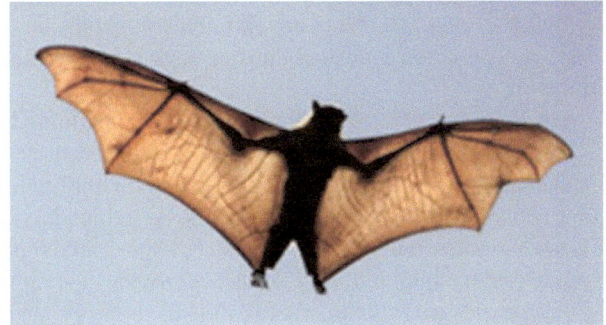

Fig. 3.19 Bats are potential carriers of the rabies virus. (Picture Source: https://www.cdc.gov/rabies. CDC)

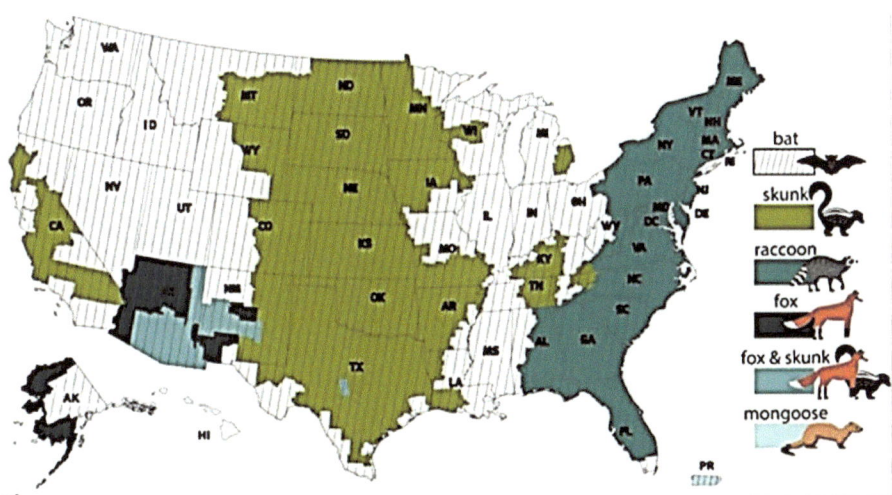

Fig. 3.20 Common mammal reservoirs of rabies by Location in the USA. (Picture Source: https://www.cdc.gov/rabies. CDC)

If a human is bitten by a domestic dog, cat or ferret, the CDC recommends that the animal be confined for 10 days of observation. If signs of infection develop, the animal should be euthanized and its brain evaluated for rabies infection and postexposure prophylaxis (PEP) initiated in the exposed person. If the domestic animal is suspected of being rabid or if the bite occurs from a wild animal that cannot be captured for observation, immediate prophylactic vaccination is generally recommended. If the biting animal's tests prove negative for rabies infection, prophylaxis can be stopped. No human rabies cases have been reported if prophylaxis is initiated within the 10-day observation window for domestic animals or if the animal's brain examination proves negative [70].

Diagnosis of rabies in animals is based on detection of the rabies virus in the affected brain, necessitating that the animal be euthanized. Most commonly, a direct fluorescent antibody test is used. With a high sensitivity and specificity, it is the "gold standard" testing method in animals, with no known cases where it failed to provide an accurate test result [70]. Histological examination of brain tissue (histopathology), immunohistochemistry and electron microscopy are other diagnostic tools.

In humans, several antemortem testing methods are available. Saliva may be tested by virus isolation or reverse transcription polymerase chain reaction (RT-PCR). Blood and serum can be tested for antibodies and skin biopsies for rabies antigens in the cutaneous nerve cells. As rabies is virtually always fatal once the virus has entered the central nervous system and the patient becomes symptomatic, postmortem examination of the brain provides a definitive diagnosis [69].

Postexposure prophylaxis (PEP) is the appropriate and urgent response to rabies exposure, as there is no treatment option once the virus has entered the central nervous system. The first line of defense is wound cleansing and debridement, independent of the relative risk for rabies. Human rabies immune globulin (HRIG) and rabies vaccine (RVA, HDCV or PCECV) are recommended on the day of rabies exposure (or as soon as possible thereafter), followed by an additional dose of vaccine on days 2, 7, and 14. Only one dose of HRIG is recommended—generally infiltrated into the bite wound and surrounding tissue at the beginning of the PEP protocol—as subsequent administration of HRIG can interfere with antibody production induced by the vaccine. If the exposed person has been previously vaccinated, only two booster doses of vaccine are recommended without immune globulin [70–72].

****

Currently, the burden of rabies disease is quite low in the USA. Approximately 5000 animal rabies cases are reported to the CDC on a yearly basis with more than 90% in wildlife—the principal reservoir being bats, raccoons, skunks, and foxes.

Fig. 3.21 Maculopapular rash of RMSF. (Picture Source: https://phil.cdc. gov. PHIL)

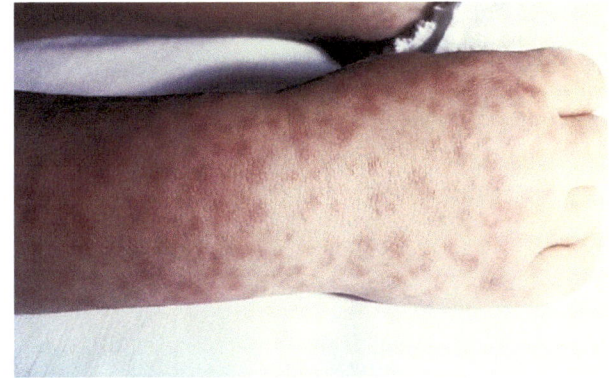

Domestic dogs represented the majority of cases in years past, before immunization was available and became law for pet dogs, cats, and ferrets in most states [70, 73].

According to the CDC, 127 human rabies cases were reported in the USA between 1960 and 2018, with approximately 25% resulting from dog bites sustained while traveling abroad. Among those cases acquired in the States, 70% were attributed to bat bites [70].

Globally, rabies causes tens of thousands of deaths per year according to the WHO [72]. Being one of the neglected tropical diseases (NTD), rabies occurs in more than 150 countries—mainly in Asia and Africa, among poor and marginalized people.[7] Of those afflicted, 40% are children under 15 years of age. The global public health costs arising from disease detection and prevention (vaccination), laboratory maintenance, animal control programs, and medical care are estimated by the WHO at $8.6 billion dollars per year [72].

Rocky Mountain Spotted Fever (*Black Measles*)

Rocky Mountain spotted fever (RMSF) is a vector-borne disease spread through the bite of a tick infected with the bacterium *Rickettsia rickettsii*. Although variable in its presentation, the disease gets its name from the characteristic rash it causes. Starting 2–4 days after the onset of fever, the rash typically begins with small red spots or blotches (maculopapular) on the wrists, forearms, and ankles (Fig. 3.21), followed by spread to the trunk and occasionally the palms and soles. Late in the disease the rash may become petechial, a sign of severe and often fatal disease [74, 75].

---

[7] The reader may find *Rabid: A Cultural History of the World's Most Diabolical Virus*, by Bill Wasik and Monica Murphy (Penguin Books: New York, NY; 2013) of interest.

Fig. 3.22 Brown dog tick
(*Rhipicephalus
sanguineus*). (Picture
Source: https://phil.cdc.
gov. PHIL)

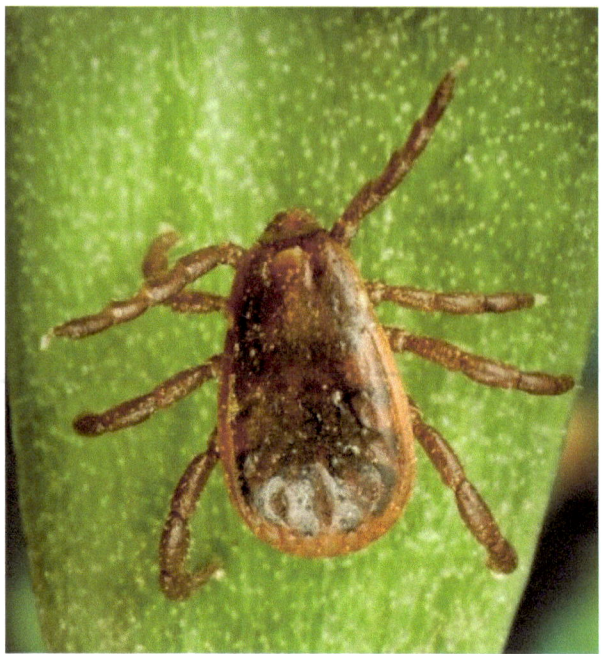

Transmission of RMSF to humans occurs through the bite of an infected tick, which is not harmed by the *Rickettsia* bacterium. Three types of ticks are known to be the principal reservoirs of RMSF bacteria [74, 75]:

- American dog ticks (*Dermacentor variabilis*) found in eastern and mid-western United States and along the Pacific Coast.
- Rocky Mountain wood tick (*Dermacentor Anderson*) found in the Rocky Mountain region.
- Brown dog tick (*Rhipicephalus sanguineus*) found worldwide.

The brown dog tick (Fig. 3.22) was identified as a disease carrier in 2003 and is now the primary vector of RMSF in the Southwest and Mexico [74]. The tick is found in and around homes wherever there are domestic dogs and appears to have a preference for humans (vs. dogs) during warm weather, raising the specter of climate-driven emergence of tick-borne diseases [76].[8] Transmission of *R. rickettsii* through blood transfusion is possible, but rare [74].

Falling within the general disease category of Spotted Fever Rickettsioses (SFR), Rocky Mountain spotted fever is a severe and rapidly progressive disease which

---

[8] The reader may find Lena H. Sun's article in *The Washington Post* (August 29, 2023/www.washingtonpost.com) of interest. The article, titled *A deadly tick-borne epidemic is raging: Dogs are the key to ending it*, spotlights with first person accounts the recent increase in RMSF cases in the southern United States and Mexico, resulting from bites from the brown dog tick.

may be fatal within days of onset without early administration of appropriate antibiotics, doxycycline being the antibiotic of choice for all ages [74, 75].

Symptoms of RMSF typically start with a sudden onset of high fever and headache 3–12 days (7 days average) after the bite of an infected tick. Additional symptoms may include nausea, vomiting, anorexia, abdominal pain, and myalgias. The prototypical maculopapular rash generally occurs 2–4 days after the onset of fever, followed by a dark petechial rash late in the course of severe disease. Late symptoms may include confusion, seizures, pulmonary compromise, limb necrosis, multiorgan failure and death [74, 77].

****

Rocky Mountain spotted fever was first recognized as a new and unique disease in 1896 in the Snake River Valley of Idaho by Army Corps physician Lt. Colonel Marshal W. Wood (1846–1933) of Boise, Idaho [78, 79]. Research on the disease began around 1900 in the Bitterroot Valley of Western Montana where residents were plagued by this deadly disease of unknown origin.

Referred to as "black measles" by local residents (Fig. 3.23), the disease had a fatality rate of nearly 4 out of 5 adult cases and was thought to result from drinking snowmelt water from the local mountains. The "black measles" moniker derived from the late appearing rash which frequently showed dark blotches or petechiae [80].

One of the first priorities of the newly incorporated Montana State Board of Health (1901) was to bring health scientists to the Bitterroot Valley to investigate the cause, treatment, and prevention of spotted fever. Among the first was Dr. Howard T. Ricketts (1871–1910) from the University of Chicago, who in 1906 demonstrated that the disease was transmitted by the bite of the Rocky Mountain wood tick and in 1906 isolated the *Rickettsia rickettsii* bacterium causing the infection [80].

Fig. 3.23 Petechial "black measles" rash of late RMSF. (Picture Source: https://www.niaid.nih.gov. NIAID)

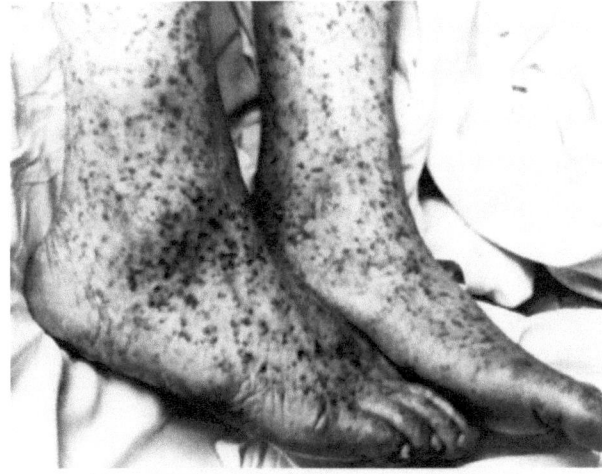

In concert with a steady rise in population density in endemic areas, there has been an ever-increasing number of cases of RMSF reported to the CDC over the years, most notably since the mid-1900s [74]. Currently (2022), there are about 6000 reported cases of RMSF in the USA each year [77]. Infections are more frequent in men than women and most commonly occur during the peak tick season of May–August, reflecting outdoor exposure risk. Despite its suggestive name, over 60% of RMSF cases are found in North Carolina, Oklahoma, Arkansas, Tennessee, and Missouri, with the exception of brown dog tick cases which are most common in the Southwest [74].

With the introduction of tetracyclines in the 1940s, the fatality rate for RMSF in the U.S. declined precipitously, but still remains around 5–10% [74]. Without prompt antibiotic therapy, death occurs in 20–30% of afflicted persons [75]. Cases are more frequent in men, but children under 10 years of age have the highest fatality rate [74].

****

The diagnosis of RMSF is principally based on the patient's clinical presentation, coupled with a history of tick exposure. Because a tick bite is painless and frequently unrecognized, a high index of suspicion is warranted when patients present with flu-like symptoms during warmer months in endemic areas. Confirmation of infection can be made with immunoglobulin (IgM and IgG) serological tests as well as polymerase chain reaction (PCR) tests and skin biopsy, as needed [75].

The *R. rickettsii* bacterium damages the endothelial cells lining blood vessels causing vasculitis and in advanced cases may cause bleeding or clotting in the brain of other vital organs. As noted previously, resultant long-term health problems may include neurological deficits, organ damage, and digit or limb necrosis requiring amputations (Fig. 3.24). There is no evidence of a persistent or chronic disease state [74].

The current preferred treatment of RMSF is with doxycycline antibiotic, which is justifiably started based on clinical suspicion alone—as the consequences of

Fig. 3.24 Digital necrosis in a hand with untreated RMSF. (Picture Source: https://www.cdc. gov. CDC)

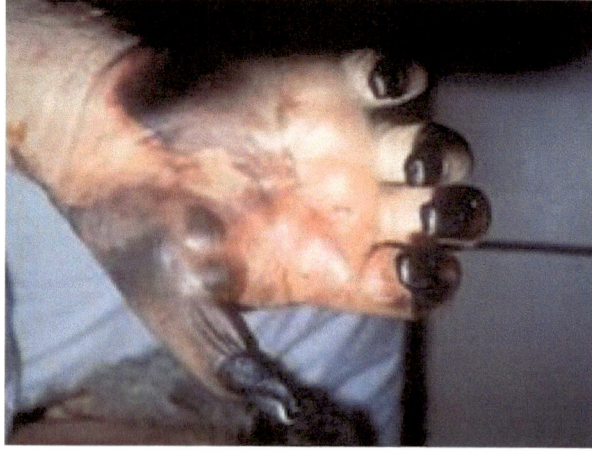

delayed treatment are potentially severe [74]. The risk of dental staining in children taking doxycycline is very low, as staining is a cumulative tetracycline dose effect and a typical treatment regimen is only for 7–10 days [75, 81]. For patients allergic to doxycycline, chloramphenicol may be recommended as an alternative drug [77].

There are no currently available vaccines for RMSF or any of the other related rickettsioses. The only protective measure is the avoidance of tick bites by staying clear of likely tick habitats (grassy, bushy areas), wearing protective clothing (long pants and shirts), treating clothing with tick repellant (permethrin), spraying exposed skin with DEET or other insect repellants, washing potentially exposed clothing with hot water, showering promptly after being outdoors, and thoroughly examining skin, gear, and pets for ticks [74].

References

Plague

1. Firth J. The history of plague—part 1. The three great pandemics. JMVH. 2012;20:2. https://jmvh.org.
2. Sun W. Plague vaccines: status and future. Adv Exp Med Biol. 2016;918:313–60. https://www.ncbi.nlm.nih.gov.
3. Wade L. From black death to fatal flu, past pandemics show why people on the margins suffer most. Science. 2020. https://www.science.org.
4. WHO. Plague. World Health Organization; 2022. https://www.who.int.
5. EyeWitness to History. The flagellants attempt to repel the black death, 1349. EyeWitness to History; 2010. https://www.eyewjtnesstohistory.com.
6. Cohn SK. Pandemics: waves of disease, waves of hate from the plague of Athens to AIDS. Hist J. 2012;85:230. https://www.ncbi.nlm.nih.gov.
7. Mark JJ. Medieval cures for the black death. World History Encyclopedia; 2020. https://www.worldhistory.org.
8. Chase M. The Barbary plague: the black death in Victorian San Francisco. New York: Random House; 2003.
9. AGN. The Late Baron Shibasaburo Kitasato. Can Med Assoc J. 1931;25(2):206. https://www.ncbi.nlm.nih.gov.
10. Hawgood BJ. Alexandre Yersin (1863-1943): discoverer of the plague bacillus, explorer and agronomist. J Med Biogr. 2008;16(3):167–72. https://pubmed.ncbi.nlm.nih.gov.
11. Simond M, Godley M, Mouriquand P. Paul-Louis Simond and his discovery of plague transmission by rat fleas: a centenary. J R Soc Med. 1998;91(2):101–4. https://pubmed.ncbi.nlm.nih.gov.
12. Randall DK. Black death at the golden gate: the race to save America from the bubonic plague. New York: W.W. Norton; 2019.
13. PBS. Bubonic plague hits San Francisco: 1900-1909. PBS—people and discoveries. 1998. https://www.pbs.org.
14. Tansey T. Plague in San Francisco: rats, racism and reform. Nature; 2019. https://www.nature.com.
15. CDC. Plague in the United States. Centers for Disease Control and Prevention; 2019. https://www.cdc.gov.
16. CDC. Plague vaccine. MMWR. 1982;31:22. https://www.cdc.gov.
17. NIH. Plague. National Institute of Allergy and Infectious Diseases; 2022. https://www.niald.nih.gov.

Yellow Fever

18. WHO. Yellow fever. World Health Organization; 2019. https://www.who.int.
19. Zhou G, Kohlhepp P, Geiser D, et al. Fate of blood meal iron in mosquitoes. J Insect Physiol. 2007;53(11):1169–78. https://www.ncbi.nlm.nih.gov.
20. CDC. Yellow fever. Centers for Disease Control and Prevention; 2022. https://www.cdc.gov.
21. Yuill TM. Yellow fever. Merck Manual: professional version. 2022. https://www.merckmanuals.com.
22. Pierce JR, Writer J. Yellow jack: how yellow fever ravaged America and Walter Reed discovered its deadly secrets. Hoboken: John Wiley & Sons, Inc; 2005.
23. Staples JE, Monath TP. Yellow fever: 100 years of discovery. JAMA. 2008;300(8):960–2. https://jamanetwork.com.
24. Prinzi A. History of yellow fever in the U.S. American Society of Microbiology. 2021. https://www.asm.org.
25. Gibson S. The yellow fever epidemic of 1878. Digital Public Library of America; 2016. https://www.dpla.org.
26. Patterson KD. Yellow fever epidemics and mortality in the United States, 1693-1905. Soc Sci Med. 1992;34(8):855–65. https://pubmed.ncbi.nlm.nih.gov.
27. CDC. Genetically modified (GM) mosquitoes. Centers for Disease Control and Prevention; 2022. https://www.cdc.gov.
28. Waltz E. Biotech firm announces results from US trial of genetically modified mosquitoes. Nature. 2022. https://www.nature.com.

Typhus

29. CDC. Typhus fevers. Centers for Disease Control and Prevention; 2020. https://www.cdc.gov.
30. CDC. Typhus fevers: information for healthcare providers. Centers for Disease Control and Prevention; 2021. https://www.cdc.gov.
31. Petri WA. Epidemic typhus. Merck Manual: professional version. 2022. https://www.merckmanuals.com.
32. Medline Plus. Typhus. National Institutes of Health/National Library of Medicine; 2020. https://medlineplus.gov.
33. Holliday TK. What an 1836 typhus outbreak taught the medical world about epidemics. Smithsonian Magazine. 2020. https://www.smithsonian.com.
34. Smith DC. Gerhard's distinction between typhoid and typhus and its reception in America, 1833-1860. Bull Hist Med. 1980;54(3):368–85. https://www.jstro.org.
35. Humphreys M. A stranger to our camps: typhus in American history. Bull Hist Med. 2006;80(2):269–90. www.pubmed.ncbi.nlm.nih.gov.
36. Raoult D. Typhus in World War I. Microbiology Society; 2014. https://microbiologysociety.org.
37. Holmes F. Typhus on the Eastern Front. University of Kansas School of Medicine; 2022. https://www.kumc.edu.
38. CDC. Typhus fevers: historical trends. Centers for Disease Control and Prevention; 2019. https://www.cdc.gov.

Malaria

39. Nosten F, Richard-Lenoble D, Danis M. A brief history of malaria. La Presse Médicale. 2022;51(3):104130. https://www.sciencedirect.com.

40. Arrow KJ, Panosian C, Gelband H. A brief history of malaria. In: Saving lives, buying time: economics of malaria drugs in an age of resistance. Washington: National Academies Press; 2004. https://www.ncbi.nlm.nih.gov.
41. PAHO. Malaria. Pan American Health Organization; 2022. https://www.paho.org.
42. CDC. Malaria. Centers for Disease Control and Prevention; 2022. https://www.cdc.gov.
43. WHO. Malaria. World Health Organization; 2022. https://www.who.int.
44. Cox FEG. History of the discovery of the malarial parasites and their vectors. Parasites Vectors. 2010;3:5. https://parasitesandvectors.biomedcentral.com.
45. Wang J, Xu C, Wong YK, et al. Artemisinin, the magic drug discovered from traditional Chinese medicine. Engineering. 2019;5(1):32–9. https://www.sciencedirect.com.
46. Laurens MB. RTS,S/AS01 vaccine (Mosquirix™): an overview. Hum Vaccin Immunother. 2020;16(3):480–9. https://www.ncbi.nlm.nih.gov.
47. Willyard C. The bumpy road to malaria vaccination. Nature. 2022;612:S48–9. https://www.nature.com.
48. WHO. WHO recommends groundbreaking malaria vaccine for children at risk: historical RTS,S/AS01 recommendation can reinvigorate the fight against malaria. Geneva: World Health Organization; 2021. https://www.who.int.
49. Gonzales SJ. Naturally acquired humoral immunity against *Plasmodium falciparum* malaria. Front Immunol. 2020;11:594653. https://www.frontiersin.org.
50. Depetris-Chauvin E, Weil DN. Malaria and early African development: evidence from sickle cell trait. Econ J. 2018;128:610. https://www.ncbi.nlm.nih.gov.
51. Bukkuri A. The history of malaria in the United States: how it spread, how it was treated, and public responses. MO J Anat Physiol. 2016;2(3):82–7. https://www.researchgate.net.
52. CDC. The history of malaria, an ancient disease. Centers for Disease Control and Prevention; 2018. https://www.cdc.gov.
53. Paltzer S. The other foe: the U.S. army's fight against malaria in the pacific theater, 1942-1945. Army Historical Foundation: National Museum of the United States Army; 2023. https://army-history.org.
54. CDC. Locally acquired cases of malaria in Florida and Texas. Centers for Disease Control and Prevention; 2023. https://www.cdc.gov.
55. Dye-Braumuller KC, Kanyangarara M. Malaria in the USA: how vulnerable are we to future outbreaks? Curr Trop Med Rep. 2021;8(1):43–51. https://www.ncbi.nlm.nih.gov.
56. Shretta R, Liu J, Cotter C, et al. Malaria elimination and eradication. In: Major infectious diseases. 3rd ed. Washington: The World Bank; 2017. https://www.ncbi.nlm.nih.gov.
57. WHO. Eliminating malaria. World Health Organization; 2023. https://www.who.int.

Dengue

58. Schaefer TJ, Panda PK, Wolford RW. Dengue fever. NCBI Bookshelf: National Library of Medicine, National Institutes of Health; 2022. https://www.ncbi.nlm.nih.gov.
59. CDC. Dengue. Centers for Disease Control and Prevention; 2022. https://www.cdc.gov.
60. Mayo Clinic. Dengue fever. Mayo Clinic; 2022. https://www.mayoclinic.org.
61. FDA. Dengvaxia. Federal Drug Administration; 2023. https://www.fda.gov.
62. Torres-Flores JM, Reyes-Sandoval A, Salazar MI. Dengue vaccines: an update. BioDrugs. 2022;36(3):325–36. https://www.ncbi.nlm.nih.gov.
63. CDC. Dengue vaccine: recommendations of the Advisory Committee on Immunization Practices, United States, 2021. Centers for Disease Control and Prevention; 2021. https://www.cdc.gov.
64. Dick OB, San Martin JL, Montoya RH, et al. The history of dengue outbreaks in the Americas. Am J Trop Med Hyg. 2012;87(4):584–93. https://www.ncbi.nlm.nih.gov.
65. CDC. Statistics and maps—2022/dengue. Centers for Disease Control and Prevention; 2023. https://www.cdc.gov.

Rabies

66. CDC. 8 zoonotic diseases shared between animals and people of most concern in the U.S. CDC Newsroom. Centers for Disease Control and Prevention; 2019. https://www.cdc.gov.
67. Scott TP, Nel LH. Lyssaviruses and the fatal encephalitic disease rabies. Front Immunol. 2021;12:786953. https://www.ncbi.nlm.nih.gov.
68. Wang J. Rabies' horrifying symptoms inspired folktales of humans turned into werewolves, vampires and other monsters. The Conversation. 2019. https://theconversation.com.
69. Rupprecht CE. Rhabdoviruses: rabies virus. 4th ed. Galveston: NCBI Bookshelf-Medical Microbiology; 1996. https://www.ncbi.nlm.nih.gov.
70. CDC. Rabies. Centers for Disease Control and Prevention; 2022. https://www.cdc.gov.
71. Cleveland Clinic. Rabies: causes, symptoms, treatment & prevention. Cleveland Clinic; 2022. https://my.clevelandclinic.org.
72. WHO. Rabies. World health Organization; 2023. https://www.who.int.
73. AVAM. Administration of rabies vaccination state laws. American Veterinary Medical Association; 2021. https://www.avma.org.

Rocky Mountain Spotted Fever

74. CDC. Rocky mountain spotted fever (RMSF). Centers for Disease Control and Prevention; 2021. https://www.cdc.gov.
75. Snowden J, Simonsen KA. Rocky mountain spotted fever (*Rickettsia rickettsii*). NCBI Bookshelf: National Library of Medicine, National Institutes of Health; 2023. https://www.ncbi.nlm.nih.gov.
76. Backus LH, López Pérez AM, Foley JE. Effect of temperature on host preference in two lineages of the brown dog tick, Rhipicephalus sanguineus. Am J Trop Hyg. 2021;104(6):2305–11. https://www.ncbi.nlm.nih.gov.
77. Cleveland Clinic. Rocky mountain spotted fever. Cleveland Clinic; 2022. https://my.clevelandclinic.org.
78. NIH. Rocky mountain spotted fever. NIH: National Institute of Allergy and Infectious Diseases; 2014. https://www.ncbi.nlm.nih.gov.
79. Filby E. Army doctor M.W. Wood and spotted fever research. South Fork Companion; 2023. https://sfcompanion.blogspot.com.
80. NIH. History of Rocky Mountain Labs (RML). NIH: National Institute of Allergy and Infectious Diseases; 2023. https://www.ncbi.nlm.nih.gov.
81. CDC. Research on doxycycline and tooth staining. Centers for Disease Control and Prevention; 2019. https://www.cdc.gov.

Chapter 4
Fecal-Oral Diseases

Abstract Fecal-oral diseases are acquired by ingesting water or food contaminated by the feces of an infected individual. Commonly, drinking water is tainted by primitive (or non-existent) sewage systems and food by using human waste for fertilizer. An infected individual can unknowingly spread fecal-oral diseases by handling food or eating/cooking utensils without appropriate handwashing following a bowel movement. Modern municipal sewer systems and sanitary water supplies have dramatically decreased the incidence of fecal-oral diseases in the United States, but they are still very common in underdeveloped countries, and Americans remain vulnerable when traveling abroad.

The fecal-oral diseases discussed in this chapter, along with their historical names and monikers, are: Cholera (*Blue Death*); Poliomyelitis (*Polio, Infantile Paralysis*); Typhoid Fever (*Bilious Fever, Burning Fever, Enteric Fever*); and Dysentery (*Bloody Flux, Montezuma's Revenge, "Trots"*).

Cholera (*Blue Death*)

Cholera is an acute diarrheal disease of the intestine caused by ingestion of water or food contaminated by the bacterium *Vibrio cholerae*. The disease has been a scourge on humanity for all time, with multiple localized epidemics and six worldwide pandemics occurring in the nineteenth century alone, killing millions worldwide. Currently, cholera causes an estimated 1.3 to 4.0 million cases and 21,000 to 143,000 deaths each year [1]. Many cases are mild and can be treated with oral hydration. More severe cases can cause death within hours due to debilitating dehydration and shock and require life-saving intravenous fluids, and in some cases antibiotics [1].

The cause is now known to be the result of direct ingestion of water or food contaminated by feces from an infected person. Eating raw or undercooked shellfish harvested from contaminated water is also a potential source of disease. The "Blue Death" moniker derives from the appearance of a patient suffering from terminal dehydration and shock (Fig. 4.1).

© The Author(s), under exclusive license to Springer Nature
Switzerland AG 2024
J. A. Shaw, *Historical Diseases from a Modern Perspective*,
https://doi.org/10.1007/978-3-031-52346-5_4

Fig. 4.1 Blue-gray
appearance of a cholera
patient. (Picture Source:
1879 French Medical Text
by Jules Rengad: *Les
grands maux et les grands
remèdes, des maladies*)

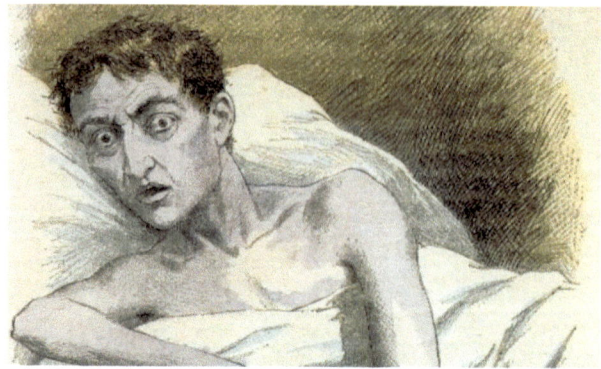

Tainted water has long been associated with cholera, dysentery, and other diseases. However, it was not until the elucidation of germ theory by Dr. Joseph Lister
(1827–1895) in his classic publications regarding antiseptic surgical technique in
The Lancet in 1867, coupled with the pioneering work of Louis Pasteur (1822–1895)
and others, did the medical community begin to suspect that bacteria were the cause
of disease. Embraced relatively quickly in Europe, germ theory took several decades
to be universally accepted by the medical community in the USA.

Interestingly, the bacterium responsible for cholera (*Vibrio cholerae*) was correctly identified by the Italian physician Filippo Pacini during an outbreak in
Florence, Italy, in 1854, long before the germ theory of disease was even proposed
or accepted. His work was ignored and/or forgotten by the scientific community and
the bacterium was independently re-discovered by Robert Koch in India in 1883 [2].

Despite credible epidemiological evidence to the contrary, as proposed by
English physician John Snow (1813–1858), it was the foul smell of the air surrounding the tainted water, not the water itself, that was felt by many to be disease causing
[3]. Known as the "miasma theory" of disease, multiple grand engineering projects
were undertaken in the mid-nineteenth century to install sewer systems to rid communities of the stench associated with stagnant sewage contaminating city streets
and rivers. For reasons not appreciated at the time, these projects greatly lessened
the incidence of cholera in many urban areas in Europe and the USA.

****

Beset with repeated epidemics of cholera, London, England, was a city in crisis in
the 1800s, with one of the worst cholera onslaughts killing over 10,000 Londoners
in 1853. The summer of 1858 was particularly hot, and the raw sewage stench—
referred to as the "Great Stink"—emanating from the River Thames and its feeding
tributaries (serving as open sewers) was overwhelming—particularly in the Houses
of Parliament, situated directly adjacent to the river (Fig. 4.2) [3–5].

With a dominant opinion that disease was spread by foul-smelling air (miasma
theory), the British Parliament rapidly approved public expenditure for a modern
sewer system to transport raw sewage into the River Thames, well downstream from

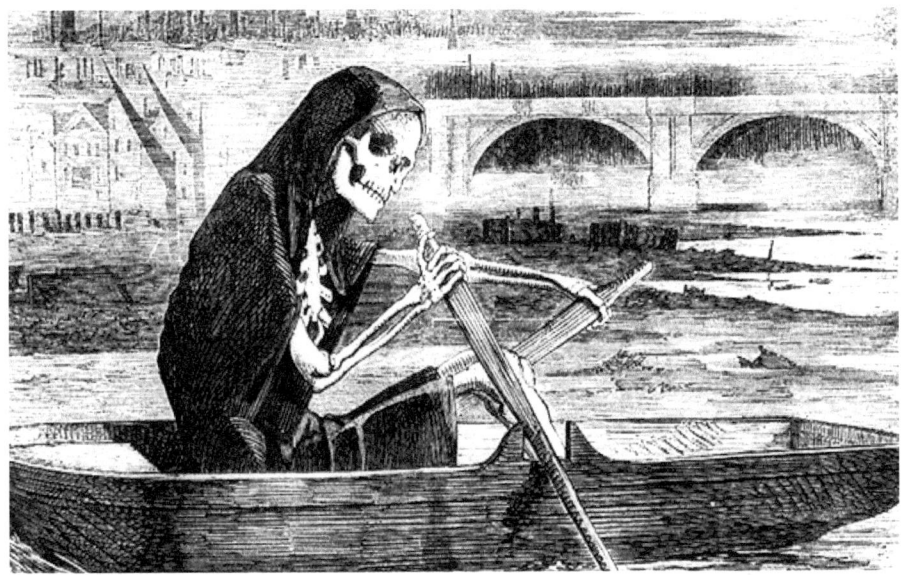

Fig. 4.2 Cartoon: *Death Rows on the Polluted River Thames*. (Picture Source: https://www.open. edu. *Punch Magazine*, 1868)

the city center. Regarded as one of the "Seven Man Made Wonders," London's sewer system was a triumph of Victorian engineering. Largely constructed between 1859 and 1868 under supervision of chief engineer Joseph Bazalgette, the initial system comprised 82 miles of intercepting sewer lines parallel to the River Thames and 1100 miles of buried street sewers. Although largely gravity fed, enormous supplemental steam-powered pumping stations were also needed to help transport sewage over uphill sections of the terrain, some honorifically named after members of the royal family [4, 5].

A more sanitary disposal method for the raw sewage was initiated in the 1880s, with only liquid waste discharged directly into the River Thames. Solids were barged and dumped out at sea. Over subsequent years, in concert with a hugely expanding population, more modern sewage treatment processes were introduced, which are in use today [5].

Similarly, as was the case with many other U.S. cities, Chicago suffered fearsome epidemics of disease during the nineteenth century, with cholera repeatedly reappearing. The *Encyclopedia of Chicago* records 1424 cholera deaths in 1854 alone, often within hours of their first symptoms. Another 210 are noted to have died from "diarrhea" and an additional 242 from "dysentery" in the same year, quite likely cases of cholera as well [6].

Like London, the city of Chicago undertook a massive reconstruction project in the mid-nineteenth century to rid the city of sewage-laden streets and miasma-related diseases. The project entailed raising many of the city's buildings and streets to accommodate a gravity-flow sewer system which emptied into the Chicago River.

Predictably, following completion of the project, the river turned into a disgusting coagulum of foul-smelling sludge, with raw human sewage combined with effluent from adjacent cattle stockyards and other industries [7].

Seemingly overlooked was the fact that the polluted river flowed into Lake Michigan, directly contaminating the city's offshore water source. After an 1863 ordinance authorized the building of a tunnel under the lake, the city of Chicago undertook another enormous project to procure uncontaminated, fresh-smelling water. The project entailed moving the city's water supply intake nearly two miles offshore, far removed from the Chicago River effluent [8, 9].

Construction of the new water intake tunnel began in 1864, in the midst of the American Civil War. By 1866, interconnecting tunnels dug 60 feet under the lake linked a huge intake crib with the city's main pumping station, which was capable of pumping 18 million gallons of water per day (Fig. 4.3) [8].

Unfortunately, of persistent concern was continued contamination of the water supply when heavy rains flooded the Chicago River and swept wastewater toward the intake crib. Cholera epidemics in 1866 and 1867 corroborated this enduring threat, and a second larger and longer lake water tunnel was dug and completed in 1874.

In a culminating step to eliminate any residual health-related concerns and, importantly, to improve the quality of the surrounding lake water, the city of Chicago undertook a final sewage disposal project in 1889. Spearheaded by the Sanitary District of Chicago, the project entailed reversing the flow of the Chicago River via a 28-mile interconnecting canal so that the city's waste would flow into the Mississippi River, not Lake Michigan. Completed in 1900, with accompanying propaganda touting "natural degradation" and "the solution to pollution is dilution"

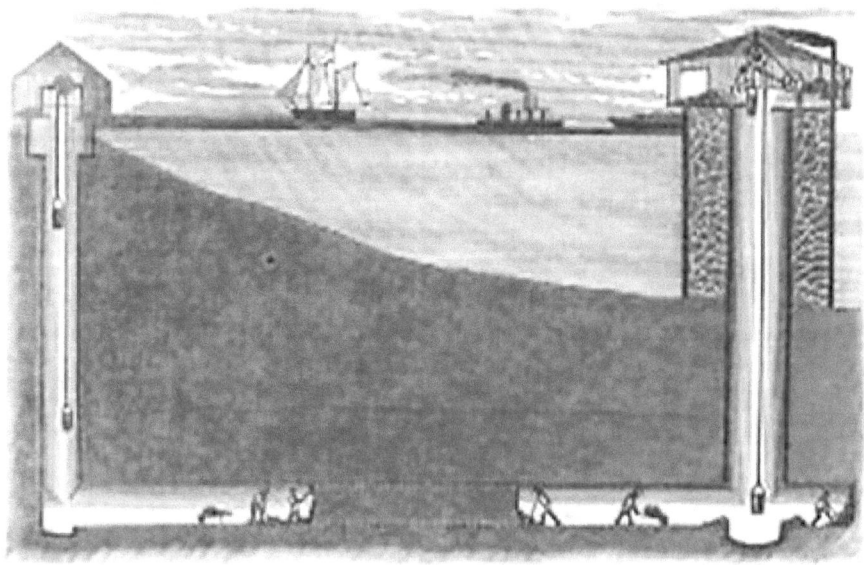

Fig. 4.3 Tunneling Chicago's water supply, 1864–1866. (Picture Source: https://www.chicago-line.com. Unidentified origin)

as sanitizing principles, the audacity of this undertaking enraged citizens of St. Louis and other downstream communities and remains a point of controversy to date [8, 9].

****

In underdeveloped countries cholera remains an endemic problem, inexorably linked to the lack of clean water and modern sanitation facilities. Peri-urban slums, displaced persons camps, and communities where floods or other natural disasters disrupt treated water supplies and sewage disposal systems are all prone to cholera outbreaks.

Three WHO prequalified oral cholera vaccines (OCV) are available globally for use in areas of endemic cholera ("hotspots") during cholera outbreaks and during humanitarian crises where contact with infected water is likely [9]. All are preferentially administered in two-dose regimens, with varying degrees of protection and duration of immunization [10]. As of 2022, more than 100 million doses of OCV have been administered during mass vaccination campaigns, according to the WHO [10].

Within the USA, routine cholera vaccination is not recommended, as the threat of water-borne cholera bacteria has been virtually eliminated by modern water and sewage treatment facilities. A single-dose oral cholera vaccine (*Vaxchora*), derived from live weakened viruses, is approved by the FDA for patients 2–64 years of age traveling to cholera-affected areas. However, as of December 2020, the manufacturer stopped production and sale of the vaccine and it is currently (2022) unavailable [11].

Poliomyelitis (*Polio, Infantile Paralysis*)

Poliomyelitis is a highly infectious viral disease transferred between people via nasal and oral secretions or, most commonly, through contact with contaminated feces or water. The virus enters the body through the mouth, multiplies in the oropharyngeal and lower gastrointestinal tract mucosa and is contagiously secreted through saliva and feces. Humans are the only natural reservoir of the disease [12, 13].

The polio virus is an enterovirus of the Picornaviridae family [14] with three wild serotypes, type 1 being the most paralytogenic and, classically, the most common cause of native polio epidemics. The disease has existed since prehistoric times, as evidenced by skeletal remains and ancient Egyptian images of children and adults with classical post-infection deformities (Fig. 4.4) [15, 16].

Affecting mostly young children under age 5, polio can attack the central nervous system, leading to extremity and respiratory paralysis, and in some cases death. However, a majority (70–75%) of people infected with polio remain completely asymptomatic. Approximately one in four patients exhibit flu-like symptoms including sore throat, fever, headache, lethargy, abdominal pain, and nausea, lasting 2–5 days. Referred to as *abortive poliomyelitis*, there are no neurologic symptoms or signs. Around 4% of patients with polio infections develop aseptic meningitis

Fig. 4.4 Ancient Egyptian engraving showing a man with a withered leg (and crutch), most likely following a polio infection. (Picture Source: https://www.cdc.gov. CDC)

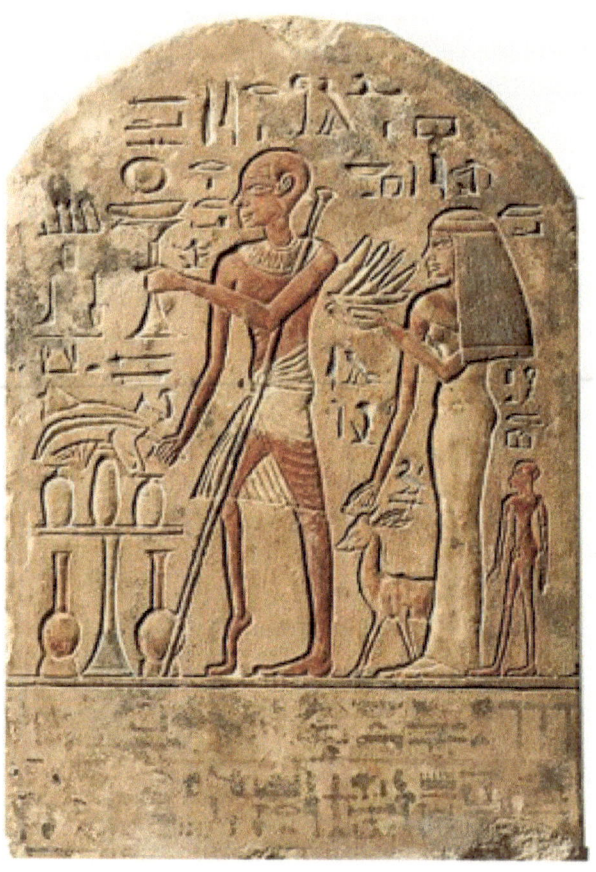

with headache and a stiff neck or back lasting 2–10 days, referred to as *nonparalytic poliomyelitis* [12, 13].

Paralytic poliomyelitis occurs when the polio virus enters the central nervous system and is characterized by skeletal muscle paralysis and, occasionally, diaphragm and intercostal muscle paralysis, affecting breathing. Accounting for less than 1% of all infections, paralytic poliomyelitis may progress very rapidly following the onset of symptoms and lead to irreversible muscle weakness or paralysis (usually in the legs) or death in a small percentage of cases. That said, most patients with paralytic affliction recover some muscle strength and function over a recuperative period of weeks to months, but two thirds are left with residual weakness[1] [12, 13, 16, 17].

The lives of many patients suffering from respiratory muscle paralysis were saved by the use of a breathing-assist device, referred to as the "iron lung." Developed in 1927 by Phillip Drinker and Louis Agassiz Shaw, the first iron lung was used at Boston Children's Hospital in 1928 to save the life of an 8-year-old girl

---

[1] The reader might enjoy Ken Dalton's autobiography *Polio and Me* (Different Drummer Press, 2016), recounting his personal experience with paralytic polio.

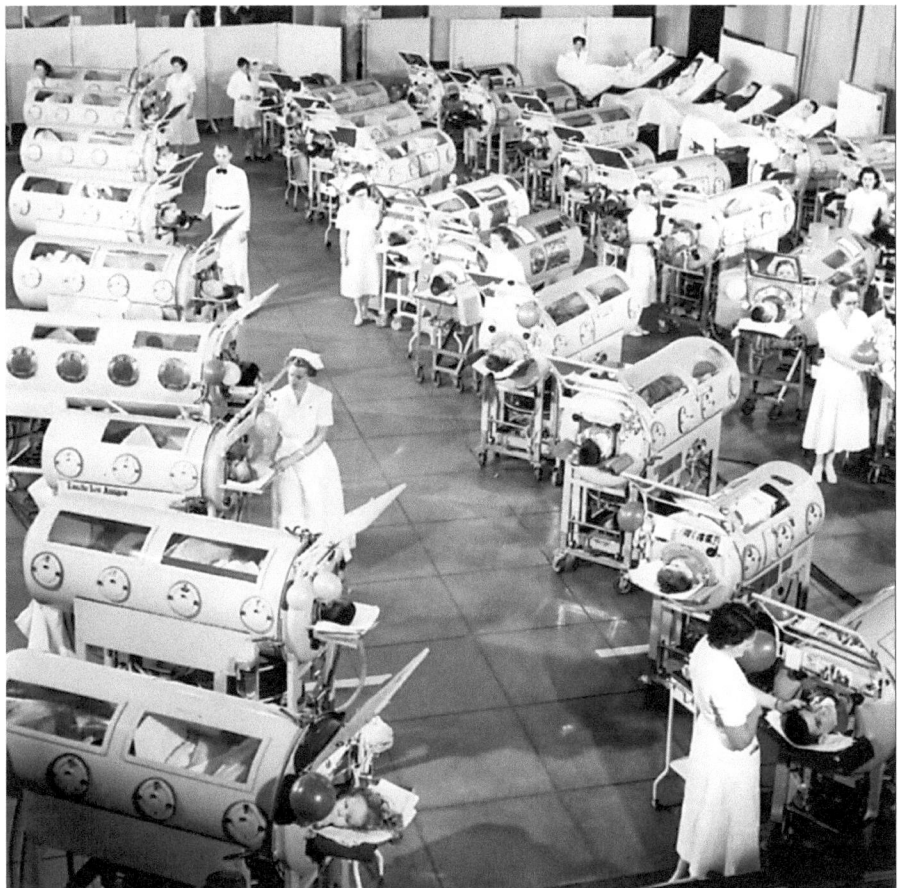

Fig. 4.5 Polio hospital "iron lung" respiratory ward, 1950. (Picture Source: https://www.journal. meddizzy.com)

with polio [18]. The body-encasing machine assisted breathing by cyclic negative pressure, causing the chest to rise and fall. Many improvements were made over the ensuing years—ultimately, with smaller chest-encasing units for hospital or home use in recovering patients. Afflicted patients were confined to an iron lung until respiratory muscle function returned sufficiently to support life, usually within 1–2 weeks after onset of paralysis (Fig. 4.5). Tragically, 5–10% paralytic patients died of irreversible pulmonary muscle paralysis [17].

Twenty to forty percent of patients develop recurrent symptoms of paralytic poliomyelitis years or decades after recovering partially or completely from their initial infection. Referred to as *post-polio syndrome*, patients may experience muscle fatigue, weakness, and atrophy to the point of becoming permanently wheelchair-bound in rare instances, even if fully functional beforehand [16, 19].

****

The first recorded outbreak of polio in the USA occurred in 1894 in Rutland County, Vermont, resulting in 18 deaths and 132 cases of permanent paralysis [20, 21]. Another outbreak in New York City in 1919 killed over 2000 persons [15]. In the late 1940s and early 1950s epidemics increased in number and size across Europe and North America, killing and disabling thousands of patients each year. The United States suffered the worst epidemic of polio in 1952, with 58,000 paralytic cases, 3145 deaths and 21,269 people crippled [21].

Many who survived the polio outbreaks suffered life-long disabilities, necessitating leg braces, crutches or wheelchairs (Fig. 4.6). Some required long-term

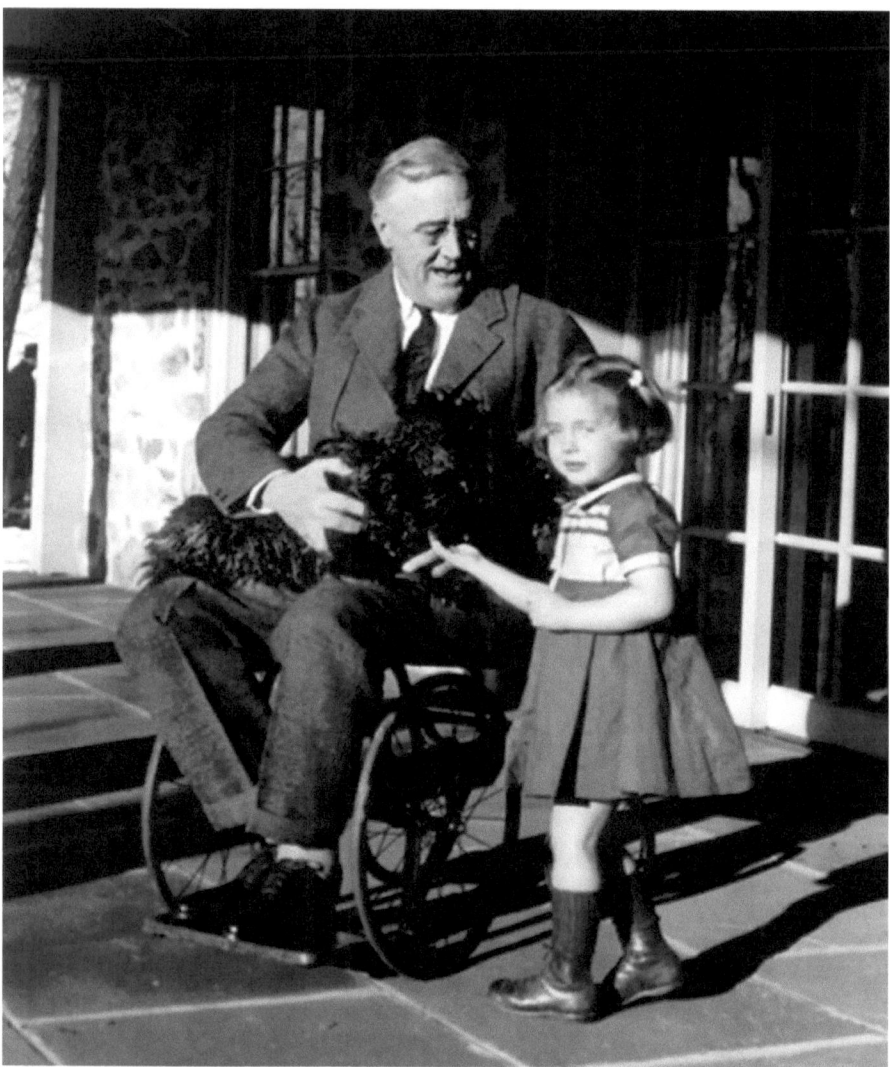

Fig. 4.6 President FDR with a young polio victim, 1941. (Picture Source: https://www. washingtonpost.com. FDR Library)

N.B.
President Franklin D. Roosevelt (1882–1945) suffered paralytic polio in 1921. He rehabilitated at Warm Springs, GA, and wore bilateral long-leg braces for the remainder of his life. He was able to stand and walk a few steps with braces and ancillary assistance and support.

breathing-assist devices if their respiratory muscles were weakened. In general, parents were terrified about disease contagion, often restricting their children's activities with friends and avoiding public gatherings, swimming pools, sports games, etc. Children were commonly shipped off to rural resident camps to escape congested cities during the warm summer months when contagion seemed most prevalent.

With worldwide cases on the rise there was an obvious need for a polio vaccine. In 1949, the polio virus was successfully cultivated in human tissue by subsequent 1945 Nobel Prize winners John Enders, Thomas Weller and Fredrick Robbins at Boston Children's Hospital [15], paving the way for vaccine development. A bitter rivalry between United States vaccine researchers, Dr. Jonas Salk (1914–1995) and Dr. Albert Sabin (1906–1993), then ensued (Fig. 4.7).

Dr. Salk developed an inactivated polio vaccine (IPV) in the early 1950s using formalin killed viruses grown on monkey kidney cells. He tested the vaccine on monkeys and later on himself and family members in 1953. Supported by the *National Foundation for Infantile Paralysis* (now known as the *March of Dimes*), a

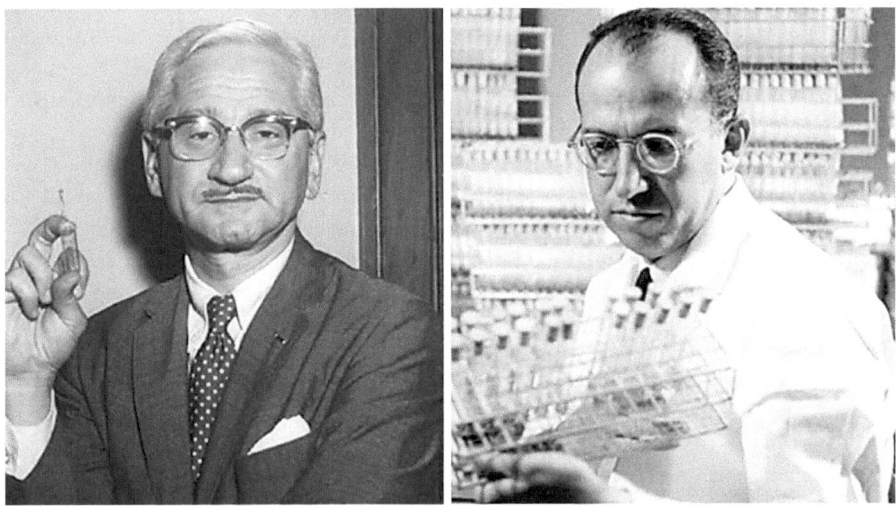

Fig. 4.7 Polio vaccine developers: Dr. Sabin (left) and Dr. Salk (right). (Pictures Source: https://aish.com. Internet)

placebo-controlled vaccination trial was carried out on 1.6 million children in Canada, Finland, and the USA [14].

The remarkably favorable study results were announced on April 12, 1955, and within hours the vaccine was approved for use in the USA. A mass vaccination program rapidly ensued, with a dramatic drop in the incidence of paralytic polio. By 1957 the annual case load decreased from 58,000 to 5600, and by 1961 only 161 cases were reported [15].[2]

An unfortunate release of inadequately inactivated vaccine viruses by the Cutter Laboratories in Berkeley, California, early in the vaccination program resulted in 260 cases of paralytic poliomyelitis and 10 deaths, casting a pall on the Salk vaccine [14]. Although modified production protocols and standards mitigated this problem, the incident, coupled with the fact that large numbers of monkeys were necessary to produce the vaccine and what appeared to be a relatively rapid decrease in protective antibody titers in vaccinated patients (necessitating serial booster shots), led the USA to transition to the competitive vaccine developed by Dr. Sabin.

Sabin's vaccine was produced from live-attenuated polio viruses and could be conveniently given orally as liquid drops or on a sugar cube. Developed in the late 1950s, the oral polio vaccine (OPV) was largely tested outside the USA due to the ongoing immunization program using the Salk vaccine in America. On the basis of these trials, coupled with the obvious advantage of oral administration, the Sabin vaccine was deemed the better of the two alternatives and, with its introduction in 1960 (licensed 1961), gradually supplanted its rival in the USA.[3] By 1968, the Salk vaccine was no longer being administered or produced in America [22].

In addition to the ease of administration, antibody testing showed that the Sabin vaccine provided a faster and longer lasting immune response. Perhaps most importantly, the vaccine offered the prospect of passive vaccination via fecal-oral transmission. While producing an immune-generating infection in the bowel, attenuated vaccine viruses excreted in feces could passively immunize others (who had not been vaccinated) by the virus' native means of fecal-oral contagion [22].

Despite what seemed to be clear advantages of the Sabin vaccine, some countries, including the Netherlands and Scandinavia, continued exclusive use of the Salk vaccine with progressive improvements in safe and efficient vaccine production using modern-day viral and cell culture techniques [22]. These improvements proved fortuitous in the long term in that mounting evidence suggested that the Sabin vaccine could lead to vaccine-associated paralytic polio (VAPP) in a small percentage of patients [14].

Be that as it may, the relative benefit-to-risk ratio continued to favor use of the Sabin vaccine throughout most of the world for many years. However, as the

---

[2] Of note: With complete philanthropic intent, Dr. Salk filed no patent claim to his vaccine. Six pharmaceutical companies were licensed to produce Salk's vaccine, with no royalty agreement or profit accrued by Dr. Salk.

[3] The author was a "Polio Pioneer," receiving the experimental Salk vaccine in 1954 (age 7) and the oral Sabin vaccine on a sugar cube in 1960 (age 12).

number of native polio cases dropped with worldwide vaccination initiatives in the 1980s and became officially eradicated in many countries in the 1990s, safety emphasis shifted to favoring the injectable Salk vaccine, once again [22].[4]

Accordingly, IPV is the only polio vaccine modality licensed for use in the USA since 2000, but OPVs continue to be used in some countries [23]. Given in isolation or in combination with other vaccines, three sequential booster shots are recommended following the initial IPV inoculation [24]. Currently, IPVs are produced for use in the USA by the pharmaceutical giants Sanofi Pasteur and GlaxoSmithKline [25].

Thanks to global vaccination initiatives, the wild poliovirus was officially eradicated across the Americas in 1997, the Western Pacific in 2000, Europe in 2002, Southeast Asia in 2014, and Africa in 2020 [20, 26]. The disease remains endemic in Afghanistan and Pakistan, but with only rare reported cases [15, 26].

That said, cases of vaccine-derived polio keep popping up, most recently in the USA in an unvaccinated person in Rockland County, New York, in August 2022. Additionally, the infecting virus was identified in the county wastewater, meeting the WHO's criteria for a circulating vaccine-derived poliovirus (cVDPV), with the obvious potential to spread disease by fecal-oral transmission [27]. As in most cases, the identified virus was a type 2 cVDPV [26, 27].

With vaccine rates dropping in the USA and other countries, the New York and other similar cases around the world have raised serious concerns referable to the spread of vaccine-derived polio [28] and have catalyzed initiatives for the development of new oral vaccines using genetically modified viruses without infective potential [29]. Although the attenuated viruses used in current OPVs only rarely cause paralytic disease, they can cause serious illness and they do pose the risk of mutation, potentially reintroducing a virulent wild polio to the global community [14]. As such, universal vaccination remains a worldwide imperative [26, 30].

Typhoid Fever (*Bilious Fever, Burning Fever, Enteric Fever*)

An ancient disease, typhoid fever is thought by many historians to be the cause of an epidemic "plague" that spread through Athens in 430 B.C.E., killing a third of the population [31]. Brought to America by the earliest colonists, infectious diseases including dysentery and typhoid decimated the Virginia colony of Jamestown (1607–1624) in a nightmarish world of recurring epidemics and early death [32]. Estimates suggest that 85% of the inhabitants of the James River colony died from typhoid between 1607 and 1624 (when the settlement was abandoned), representing over 6000 inhabitants [33]. With no prior exposure/immunity to these

---

[4]The reader may find *The Washington Post* interactive web page, *The history of polio and the vaccines that nearly eradicated it,* by Ruby Mellen (Aug 20, 2022) of interest (www.washington-post.com).

pathogens—referred to as a "virgin soil disease"—indigenous people suffered large scale outbreaks, as well [33].

Abigail Adams (1744–1818) died of typhoid fever [34] as did thousands of other early Americans crowded into cities with primitive or non-existent water supply and/or waste disposal infrastructures. Two thirds of Civil War soldiers died from infectious diseases, prominent among them being typhoid fever. Poor sanitation practices and a general lack of knowledge regarding germ theory led to 75,148 documented cases of typhoid within the Union army and 27,058 deaths (36% mortality rate), with an equivalent incidence likely within the Confederate army [35]. Similarly, typhoid fever was the major killer of American soldiers during the Spanish-American War (1898). Proving more deadly than the Cuban battlefields, 20,738 soldiers contracted the disease and 1590 died (7.7% mortality) in the 4-month long war [36].

Without question, the infamous case of Mary Mallon (1869–1938) brought typhoid fever to the forefront of America's consciousness.[5] After emigrating to the USA from Ireland in 1884, Mallon settled into a career as a domestic cook for a number of wealthy New York families. Following the 1906 outbreak of typhoid within the Charles Warren family, for whom she was working, Ms. Mallon was identified as the first known asymptomatic carrier of an infectious disease by sanitation engineer George Soper [37].

With numerous typhoid outbreaks traced to kitchens where she worked, corroborated by positive stool cultures for the bacillus known to cause typhoid, Mary was forcibly quarantined on New York's North Brother Island in 1907. Branded by the press as "Typhoid Mary" (Fig. 4.8), she remained quarantined for 3 years until her release back into society in 1910 with a strict order not to seek employment in commercial cooking. Violating that order, Mallon began cooking for Sloane Maternity Hospital in Manhattan several years later under the assumed name of "Mary Brown." Within several months of her employment at least 25 people at the hospital became ill with typhoid, with two deaths [37].

In 1915 Mallon was re-committed to North Brother Island, where she spent the rest of her life until her death in 1938. According to Soper's 1939 report in the *Bulletin of the New York Academy of Medicine* [38], 53 known typhoid cases were traced to Mary Mallon, with three deaths.

****

Following the pioneering work of other clinicians, Karl Joseph Ebert (1835–1926) is credited with definitively identifying the bacterium responsible for typhoid fever in 1879 (published 1980) by isolating the bacterium from typhoid patients while failing to identify the same bacterium in comparative patients suffering from other diseases [37]. Today, the bacillus goes by the scientific name *Salmonella enterica* serotype typhi (commonly shortened to *Salmonella typhi*) and is a flagellated gram-negative rod (Fig. 4.9) whose only reservoir is the human body [39]. Other

---

[5]The reader might be interested in the historical novel, *Fever*, by Mary Beth Keane (Scribner: New York, NY; 2014) based on the life of Mary Mallon and/or the excellent video depicting Mallon's life at: https://www.news-medical.net/health/typhoid-fever-history.aspx.

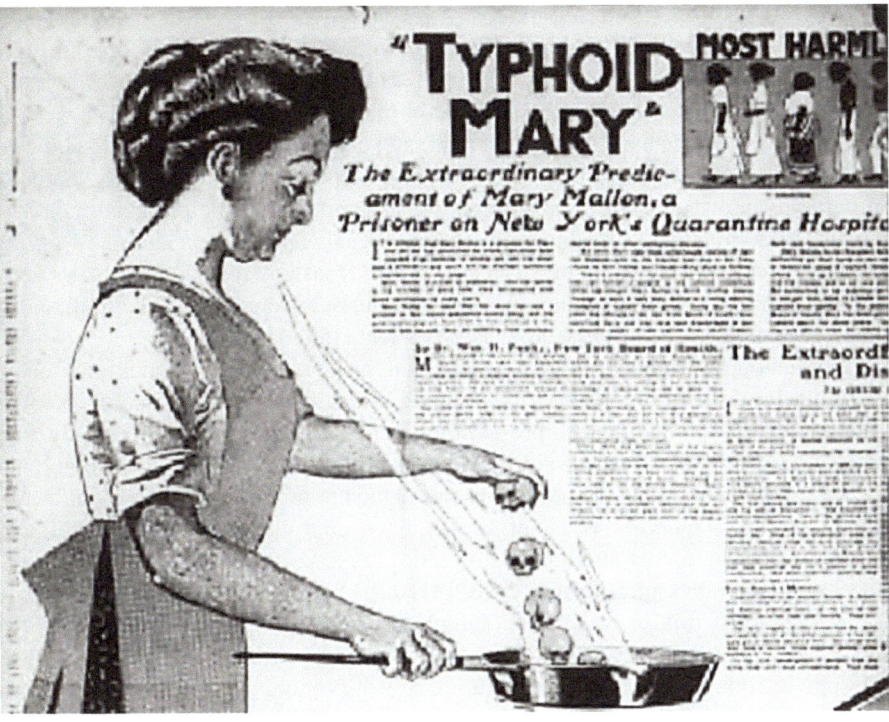

Fig. 4.8 "Typhoid Mary," as depicted in a newspaper of the time. (Picture Source: https://www.gavi.org. New *York American*, 1909)

Fig. 4.9 CDC rendering of *Salmonella enterica*. (Picture Source: https://www.asm.org. CDC: Public Health Image Library)

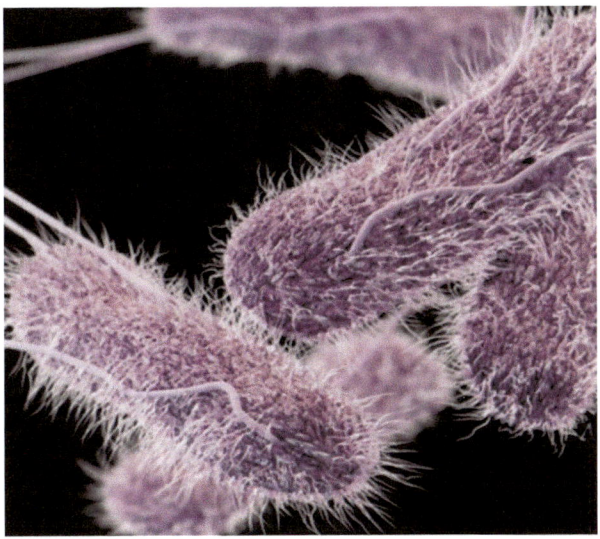

Salmonella serotypes, referred to as *Salmonella paratyphi* (A, B, C), are also now known to cause typhoid-like symptoms (paratyphoid fever), but generally of milder severity and with a lower mortality rate [40, 41].

The symptoms of typhoid fever include prolonged fever (lasting 3–4 weeks), fatigue, headache, nausea, abdominal pain, and constipation or diarrhea [41]. Fever usually starts about 1 week after ingestion of the infecting organism and classically progresses in a "stepladder" fashion with peaks and troughs before becoming sustained. Abdominal pain and distention (hepatomegaly and splenomegaly) of varying degrees are seen in all patients. Occasionally, transient rose-colored spots may appear on the trunk or abdomen. An incongruously lowered pulse rate in the presence of fever (Faget sign) is seen in some patients [39–41].

Confusion, delirium, intestinal perforation, and hemorrhagic shock may occur within a few weeks of symptom onset, with a resultant mortality rate of 12–30% among typhoid patients in the pre-antibiotic era [42]. Currently, with timely supportive care and antibiotic therapy, the mortality rate is 1–4% [43]. Fluoroquinolones or third-generation cephalosporins are the mainstay of antibiotic treatment at this time, but ever-emerging resistant strains have complicated treatment regimens necessitating the use of alternative antibiotics (e.g., azithromycin or carbapenems) or combination therapies in some cases [41, 42].

A generally milder relapse of symptoms occurs in approximately 10% of untreated patients, typically 1–3 weeks after recovery from the original infection. Despite adequate antibiotic therapy, up to 5% of typhoid patients become chronic carriers of *Salmonella typhi*, excreting the bacterium in their stool or urine for more than 1 year after recovering from an acute infection [39, 42]. Cholecystectomy may be curative if gallstones accompany a carrier state [41].

Typhoid fever (and paratyphoid fever) is acquired through the ingestion of food or water contaminated with the feces of people who are actively infected with the disease, or are chronic carriers. Inadequate sewage and drinking water infrastructures (Fig. 4.10) make the disease most common in third-world countries such as India, Bangladesh, and Pakistan. Inadequate hand washing after defecation is another mode of transmission, most notably during food preparation by asymptomatic carriers.

The CDC estimates that between 11 and 21 million cases of typhoid fever, with 2000 deaths, occur annually throughout the world. Added to that, they estimate that five million cases of paratyphoid fever occur yearly [42].

Currently, the risk of infection with typhoid is very low in the USA (Fig. 4.11). With passage of the Pure Food and Drug Act in 1906, coupled with improvements in municipal sewage disposal, drinking water disinfection, sanitation practices, refrigeration, and pasteurization, the incidence of food and water-borne diseases began to markedly diminish in the early twentieth century [44].[6] Although unreported or undiagnosed cases may make the actual incidence much higher, about 350

---

[6] The reader might enjoy *The Jungle* by Upton Sinclair (Seawolf Press, 1906), a very influential book depicting the unsanitary working conditions in the meat- packing industry.

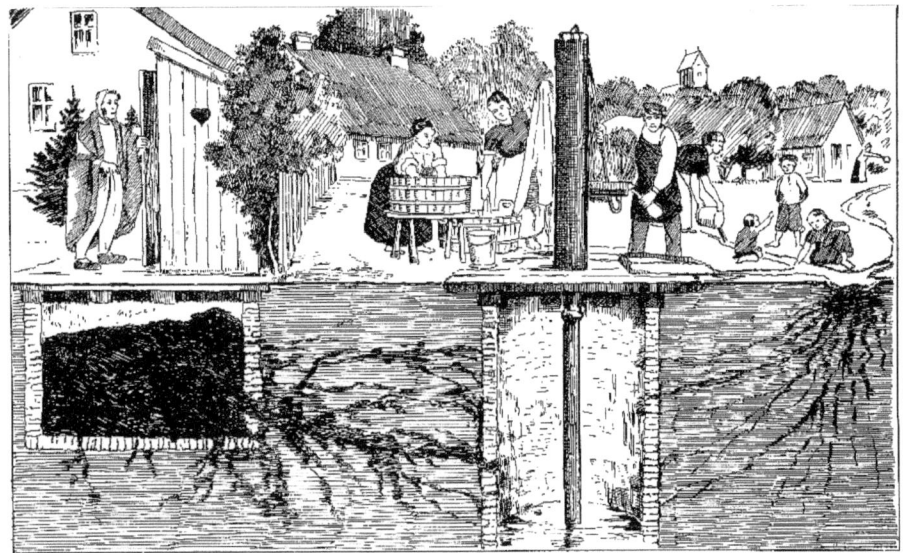

Fig. 4.10 1939 illustration of fecal drinking water contamination modalities. Unidentified illustrator. (Picture Source: www.en.wikipedia.org. *Vore Sygdome*; Bind II, side 116)

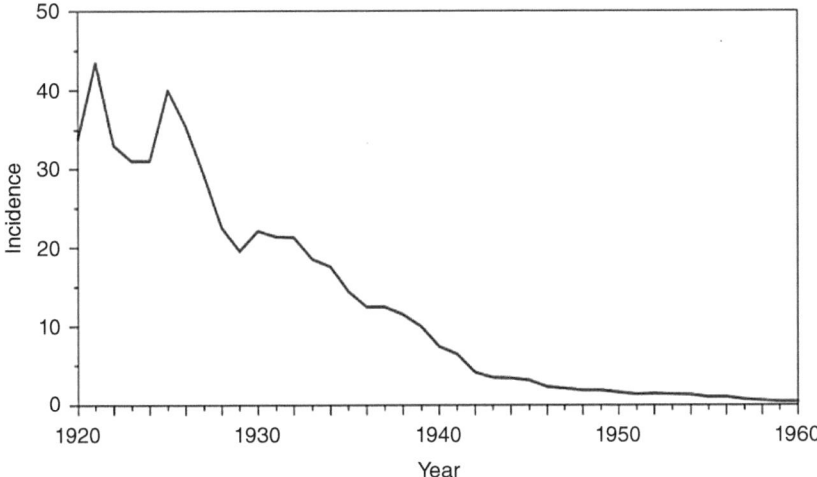

*Per 100,000 population.

U.S. DEPARTMENT OF HEALTH & HUMAN SERVICES

Fig. 4.11 Incidence of typhoid fever in the USA: 1920–1960. (Picture Source: https://www.cdc.gov. CDC)

patients are currently diagnosed with typhoid fever and 90 patients with paratyphoid fever annually in the USA, according to the CDC [42]. Most patients report recent travel to countries where these diseases are common.

****

The diagnosis of typhoid fever is based on the patient's clinical presentation (fever, abdominal pain, constipation or diarrhea), coupled with a history of residing in or traveling to an endemic area. Confirmatory *Salmonella typhi* (or *paratyphi*) bacterial cultures from stool, blood or bone marrow clinches the diagnosis. Serological testing for *Salmonella* antibodies (Widal's test) may be helpful but is notoriously unreliable due to cross reactivity with other *Salmonella* species (false positive result) and a low sensitivity (false negative result). Other diagnostic modalities, including punch biopsy of skin rose spots and polymerase chain reaction (PCR) tests, are also available [40, 41].

British bacteriologist Almroth Edward Wright (1861–1947) is generally credited with the development of the first typhoid fever vaccine in 1896. Using heat-killed typhoid bacilli, the vaccine was used successfully among British soldiers during the South African (Boer) War and WW I [45]. Currently, two typhoid vaccines are available in the USA and used widely throughout the world, according to the WHO [46]. One is an injectable vaccine based on a purified bacterial antigen, approved for persons over 2 years of age. The second is a live-attenuated oral vaccine for persons aged over 6 years. Additionally, a new typhoid conjugate vaccine with a longer lasting protective immunity was prequalified by the WHO in 2017 for children over 6 months of age [46].

Vaccination is recommended by the WHO for travelers destined for endemic typhoid areas. Importantly, the WHO recommends the following universal precautions to world travelers [46]:

• Ensure food is properly cooked and hot when served.
• Drink only pasteurized or boiled milk.
• If of questionable origin, boil or disinfect drinking water.
• Avoid ice unless it is made from treated water.
• Wash hands thoroughly and frequently.
• Wash fruits and vegetables, preferably eating only those that can be peeled.

Dysentery (*Bloody Flux, Montezuma's Revenge, "Trots"*)

Dysentery is an infectious gastroenteritis characterized by copious diarrheal stools containing mucus and blood. Although a variety of bacteria, viruses, and parasites can cause diarrhea, there are two main causes of dysentery:

1. Bacillary dysentery or shigellosis is caused by Shigella bacteria (Fig. 4.12) and is the principal type of dysentery found in the USA. First identified by Kiyoshi

Fig. 4.12 Shigella bacteria depiction. (Picture Source: https://www.cdc.gov/shigella. CDC)

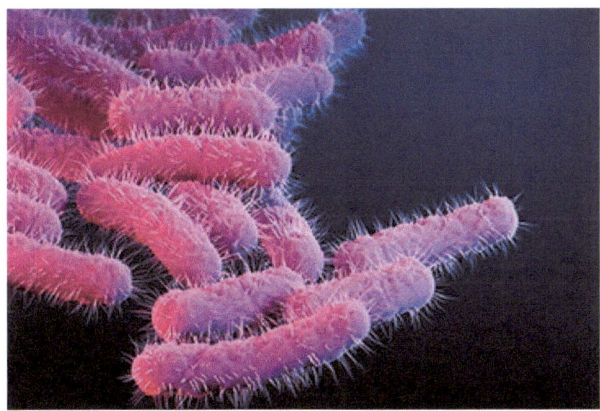

Shiga (1871–1957) in 1898 [47], there are four Shigella species known to cause dysentery, the *Shigella sonnei* species being the most common infecting species in the States. *Shigella dysenteriae* type 1 causes the most severe symptoms and is the deadliest, but is rare in America [48].

2. Amebic dysentery or amebiasis is caused by a single-celled ameba parasite called *Entamoeba histolytica*. The parasite is mainly found in tropical areas and is *principally contracted* abroad or brought to the States by immigrants [49].

Both types of dysentery are spread by fecal-oral communication via contaminated drinking water or eating food prepared by an infected person who has not washed his or her hands adequately after a bowel movement. Hand-to-mouth contagion after touching any fecally contaminated surface or coming in oral contact with stool during sexual activity are additional ways of transmission [48, 49].

Most persons with Shigella infections experience profuse (near-liquid) diarrhea flecked with blood and mucus lasting more than 3 days, often accompanied by fever, nausea and vomiting, and abdominal pain or cramps. Symptoms start 1–2 days after infection and last, on average, around 7 days. Complications include inflammatory colon dilation and kidney failure. Copious loss of bodily fluids can result in death. Most vulnerable are children, the elderly, and the immunocompromised [48, 50, 51].

Infection with *E. histolytica* may cause no or only mild symptoms including loose stools and abdominal pain or cramping. However, a severe form, referred to as amebic dysentery, produces symptoms similar to shigellosis. Parasite spread to the liver can cause abscess formation and parasitic intestinal ulcerations may lead to bowel perforation and death. Rarely, parasites may spread through the blood to the brain, lungs, or other organs [49, 51].

The diagnosis of dysentery is made by presenting symptoms, exposure history, and stool microscopy or culture for parasites or bacteria, depending on the type of infection. Antibody tests may be helpful, as well. Diagnostic confusion is often rendered by *Entamoeba dispar* which is a very common parasite and appears identical under the microscope to *E. histolytica*. *E. dispar* is harmless and does not require treatment but is frequently assumed to be *E. histolytica* and treated anyway to avoid any possible diagnostic/treatment errors [49, 51].

Treatment of dysentery principally consists of oral or intravenous hydration, as clinically indicated. Blood transfusions may be necessary in rare cases. That said, most cases of bacillary dysentery resolve on their own without formal treatment; but, if severe, may necessitate antibiotic (ciprofloxacin or ceftriaxone) therapy in addition to aggressive fluid resuscitation. Amebiasis is generally treated with antimicrobials such as metronidazole (Flagyl) or paromomycin in addition to symptomatic treatment [48, 49, 52].

Bismuth subsalicylate (*Pepto-Bismol*) may be preventatively helpful in some people, but antidiarrheal medications such as loperamide (Imodium) should be avoided (or only used short term), as they hinder shedding the causative organisms in the stool. There are currently no vaccines for dysentery of either type [48, 51].

****

Without question, dysentery arrived with colonists to America in the 1600–1700s [53]. Conditions were ideal for spread, with pervasive indifference to personal hygiene and unsanitary disposal of human waste on immigrant ships, and in early settlements and soldier encampments. With limited or no understanding of infectious diseases and their modes of transmission (and, of course, no antibiotics or intravenous fluids), patients were often treated with bloodletting, blistering, and ingestion of purgatives and emetics [54]. Ultimately, all had to let the disease run its course, with many dying from severe dehydration.

In the Mexican War there were a total of 12,535 war deaths, 10,986 due to infectious diseases with dysentery representing the overwhelming majority [55]. Disregard for personal hygiene and sanitary waste disposal fueled the outbreaks, draining resources, impacting preparedness, and eroding troop morale in the process.

During the Civil War, army camps were breeding grounds of disease, and sickness was an ever-present companion of soldiers on both sides of the conflict. Commonly referred to as "the runs" or "the flux" or "the trots," there were 1,900,000 reported cases of dysentery or diarrhea among the 2 million men who served in the Union army [56]. With limited understanding of the origins of disease, no distinction was made between "diarrhea" (a symptom) and "dysentery" (a disease). Be that as it may, thousands of Civil War troops died from bowel disorders or were discharged to home with chronic diarrhea. Many others were rendered susceptible to other diseases with a weakened state of health. Soldiers suffering with diarrhea were commonly treated with whiskey or with purgatives such as turpentine or castor oil, which, in retrospect, probably further inflamed the bowels [56, 57].

Life in the trenches of WWI, with no facilities to bathe or wash hands and no provisions to dispose of excreta while under fire, meant that soldiers often survived in ankle-deep sewage-laden filth. Bacillary dysentery was endemic and epidemic [58].

In WWII, frequent dysentery outbreaks occurred among allied troops operating in Burma, the Far East, and North Africa. Army medical records indicate that there were 523,331 reported cases among U.S. troops between 1942 and 1945 [59]. Although of limited significance with respect to mortality, diarrheal disorders were a major cause of morbidity and ineffectiveness among troops [59]. Of particular notoriety was the scourge of dysentery in Japanese POW camps (Fig. 4.13) [60].

Currently (2022), the CDC estimates that there are 450,000 Shigella infections each year in the USA, accounting for an estimated $93 million in direct medical costs. As is the case with many infectious diseases, one of the major concerns is evolving antimicrobial resistance [48].

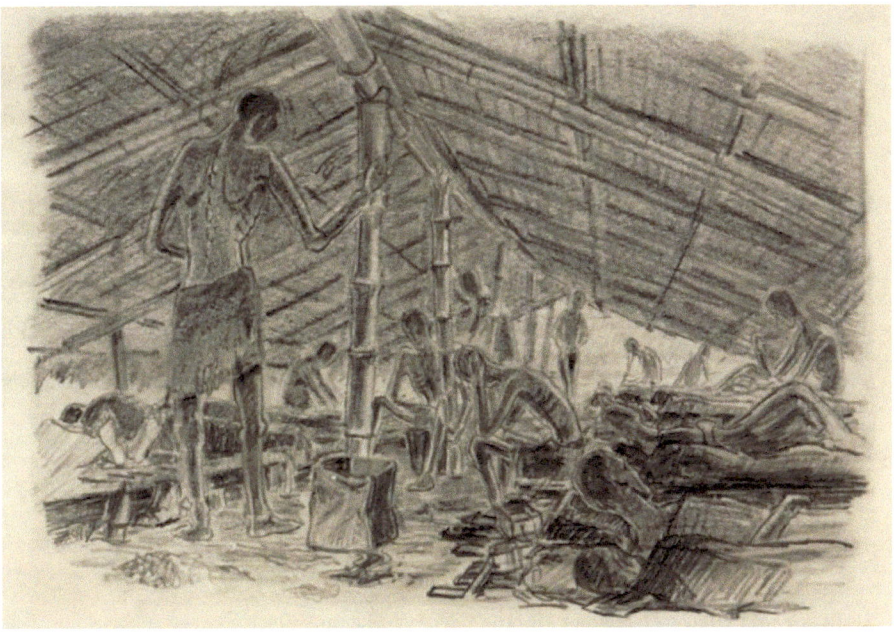

Fig. 4.13 Allied POWs with dysentery in a Japanese camp in Thailand, 1943. Unidentified Artist. (Picture Source: https://en.wikipedia.org. Imperial War Museums, UK)

References

Cholera

1. WHO. Cholera. Geneva: World Health Organization; 2021. https://www.who.int.
2. Carboni GP. The enigma of Pacini's *Vibrio cholerae* discovery. J Med Microbiol. 2021;70(11):1450. https://pubmed.ncbi.nlm.nih.gov.
3. Begum F. Mapping disease: John Snow and cholera. London: Royal College of Surgeons of England; 2016. https://www.reseng.ac.uk.
4. BBC. Seven man made wonders. London sewers. British Broadcasting Corporation; Undated. https://www.bbc.co.uk/england.
5. Everett B. How London got its Victorian sewers. The Open University; 2018. https://open-learnmedium.edu.
6. Nugent W. Epidemics. Encyclopedia of Chicago. Chicago Historical Society; 2005. https://www.encyclopedia.chicagohistory.org.
7. Chicagology. 1855-raising Chicago. Chicagology. 1855. https://chicgology.com.
8. Sheahan JW. The Chicago "Crib". Chicago Illustrated; 1866. https://chicagology.com.
9. Smithers GD. Reversing a river: how Chicago flushed its human waste downstream. We're History. 2020. https://werehistory.org.
10. WHO. Cholera. Geneva: World Health Organization; 2022. https://www.who.int.
11. CDC. Cholera-*Vibrio cholerae* infection: vaccines. Centers for Disease Control and Prevention; 2022. https://www.cdc.gov.

Poliomyelitis

12. Tesini BL. Poliomyelitis. Merck Manual: professional version. 2022. https://www.merckmanuals.com.
13. PAHO. The history of polio—from eradication to re-emergence. Washington: Pan American Health Organization; 2022. https://www.paho.org.
14. Baicus A. History of polio vaccination. World J Virol. 2012;1(4):108–14. https://www.ncbi.nlm.nih.gov.
15. WHO. History of polio: a crippling and life-threatening disease. Geneva: World Health Organization; 2022. https://www.who.int.
16. CDC. What is polio? Centers for Disease Control and Prevention; 2022. https://www.cdc.gov.
17. WHO. Poliomyelitis. Geneva: World Health Organization; 2022. https://www.who.int.
18. Science Museum. The iron lung. Science Museum; 2018. https://www.sciencemuseum.org.uk.
19. CDC. Post-polio syndrome. Centers for Disease Control and Prevention; 2021. https://www.cdc.gov.
20. Flo Health. Polio vaccination history: timeline of poliomyelitis discovery and vaccine invention. Flo Health; 2021. https://flo.health.
21. Fuchs M, Zundel J. Polio vaccine: history and inventor. Study.com. 2022. https://study.com.
22. Blume S, Geesink I. A brief history of polio vaccines. Science. 2000;288:5471. https://www.science.org.
23. CDC. Polio vaccination: what everyone should know. Centers for Disease Control and Prevention; 2022. https://www.cdc.gov.
24. CDC. Polio vaccination in the US. Centers for Disease Control and Prevention; 2022. https://www.cdc.gov.
25. CDC. Vaccines and immunizations: U.S. vaccine names. Centers for Disease Control and Prevention; 2019. https://www.cdc.gov.

26. KFF. The U.S. government and global polio efforts. KFF; 2022. https://www.kff.org.
27. CDC. The United States confirmed as country with circulating vaccine-derived poliovirus. Centers for Disease Control and Prevention; 2022. https://www.cdc.gov.
28. Nature Editorial. Vaccine-derived polio is undermining the fight to eradicate the virus. Nature. 2023;618(7965):434. https://www.nature.com.
29. Yeh TM, Smith M, Carlyle S, et al. Genetic stabilization of attenuated oral vaccines against poliovirus types 1 and 3. Nature. 2023;619:135–42. https://www.nature.com.
30. CDC. Who we are: CDC and the global polio eradication initiative. Centers for Disease Control and Prevention; 2013. https://www.cdc.gov.

Typhoid

31. Martin CS. The plague of Athens killed tens of thousands, but its cause remains a mystery. National Geographic; 2021. https://www.nationalgeographic.com.
32. Earle C. Environment, disease and mortality in early Virginia. J Hist Geogr. 1979;5(4):365–90. https://www.sciencedirect.com.
33. Hagen A. The toxin-based diseases common in North America during the 1600-1700s. Washington: American Society of Microbiology; 2019. https://www.asm.org.
34. NPS. Abigail Adams (1744-1818). National Park Service; 2015. https://www.nps.gov.
35. Mahr M. Typhoid fever—one of the civil war's deadliest diseases. National Museum of Civil War Medicine; 2021. https://www.civilwarmed.org.
36. Cirillo VJ. Fever and reform: the typhoid epidemic in the Spanish-American War. J Hist Med Allied Sci. 2000;55(4):363–97. https://muse.jhu.edu.
37. Marineli F, Tsoucalas G, Karamanou M, Androutsos G. Mary Mallon (1869-1938) and the history of typhoid fever. Ann Gastroenterol. 2013;26(2):132–4. https://www.ncbi.nlm.nih.gov.
38. Soper GA. The curious career of Typhoid Mary. Bull N Y Acad Med. 1939;15(10):698–712. https://www.ncbi.nlm.nih.gov.
39. Ashurst JV, Truong J, Woodbury B. Salmonella typhi. In: StatPearls. New York: National Institutes of Health; 2022. https://www.ncbi.nlm.nih.gov.
40. Maskalyk J. Typhoid fever. Can Med Assoc J. 2003;169(2):132. https://www.ncbi.nlm.nih.gov.
41. Bhandari J, Thada PK, DeVos E. Typhoid fever. In: StatPearls. New York: National Institutes of Health; 2022. https://www.ncbi.nlm.nih.gov.
42. CDC. Typhoid fever and paratyphoid fever: information for healthcare professionals. Centers for Disease Control and Prevention; 2021. https://www.cdc.gov.
43. Kim SH, Bansai J. A rare case of typhoid fever in the United States associated with travel to Mexico. Cureus. 2022;14(2):e22316. https://www.ncbi.nlm.nih.gov.
44. CDC. Achievements in public health, 1900–1999: safer and healthier foods. MMWR. 1999;48:40. https://www.cdc.gov.
45. Editors Encyclopedia Britannica. Sir Almroth Edward Wright: British bacteriologist and immunologist. Encyclopedia Britannica: Update; 2022. https://www.britannica.com.
46. WHO. Typhoid. World Health Organization; 2018. https://www.who.int.

Dysentery

47. Trofa AF, Ueno-Olsen H, Oiwa R, et al. Dr. Kiyoshi Shiga: discoverer of the dysentery bacillus. Clin Infect Dis. 1999;29(5):1303–6. https://academic.oup.com.cid.
48. CDC. Shigella—shigellosis. Centers for Disease Control and Prevention; 2023. https://www.cdc.gov.

49. CDC. Parasites—amebiasis—*Entamoeba histolytica* infection. Centers for Disease Control and Prevention; 2021. https://www.cdc.gov.
50. Dejkam A, Hatam-Nahavadi K. Dysentery in children. Iran J Public Health. 2021;50(9):1930–1. https://www.ncbi.nlm.nih.gov.
51. MediResource. Dysentery. MediResource, Inc.; 2023. https://medbrodcast.com.
52. Traa BS, Walker CLF, Munos M, et al. Antibiotics for the treatment of dysentery in children. Int J Epidemiol. 2010;39(1):70–4. https://www.ncbi.nlm.nih.gov.
53. ASM. The toxin-based diseases common in North America during the 1600-1700s. American Society of Microbiology; 2019. https://asm.org.
54. Parascandola J. Drug therapy in colonial and revolutionary America. Am J Hosp Pharm. 1976;33(8):807–10. https://pubmed.ncbi.nlm.nih.gov.
55. Cirillo VJ. "More fatal than powder and shot": dysentery in the U.S. Army during the Mexican War, 1846-48. Perspect Biol Med. 2009;52(3):400–13. https://pubmed.ncbi.nlm.nih.gov.
56. Robertson J. The dysentery enemy. Radio WVTF; 2019. https://www.wvtf.org.
57. Backus PG. Common diseases of the 18th and 19th century. American Battlefield Trust; 2022. https://www.battlefields.org.
58. Wright DJ, Drasar B. Dysentery in World War I: *Shigella* a century on. The Lancet. 2014;385:9955. https://www.thelancet.com.
59. AMEDD Center of History & Heritage. Army experience with diarrheal disorders during World War II. Army Medical Department of the U.S. Army; Undated. https://achh.army.mil.
60. Robson D, Welch E, Beeching NJ, et al. Consequences of captivity: health effects of far east imprisonment in World War II. QJM. 2008;102(2):87–96. https://academic.oup.com.

Chapter 5
Sexually Transmitted Diseases

Abstract Sexually transmitted diseases are communicated with the exchange of bodily fluids during sexual intercourse or by intimate contact with an open lesion (sore) associated with a particular disease. Sexually transmitted diseases have been a scourge on society for centuries and have afflicted Americans most prominently during periods of war, severely affecting troop strength and preparedness during the Civil War, WWI and WWII. A truly effective treatment was not available until the development of penicillin, which became obtainable toward the end of WWII. Currently, sexually transmitted diseases are on the rise in the United States, partly due to an increase of sex between men. Additionally, the incidence of congenital syphilis has risen dramatically in recent years.

The sexually transmitted diseases discussed in this chapter, along with their historical names and monikers, are: Syphilis (*French Pox, Great Pox, "Bad Blood"*) and Gonorrhea (*"The Clap," "The Drip"*).

Syphilis (*French Pox, Great Pox, "Bad Blood"*)

The origin of pandemic syphilis remains controversial, to date [1]. Some surmise that isolated pockets of syphilis existed throughout Europe, Asia, and the Americas since prehistoric times, but remained confined in scope and distribution by social and geographic isolation, or was simply not recognized as a unique disease. Spread of disease occurred with increasing population density, changing lifestyles, migrating traders and refugees, warfare, and changing sexual mores.

The "Columbian Exchange" school of thought suggests that Columbus and his men brought the disease back from the Americas, reflecting a new world order where communicable diseases, such as smallpox and syphilis, were transmitted and spread by expanding intercontinental exploration, trade, and travel.

Although somewhat controversial, the New World theory of origin is supported by clear evidence of treponematosis in skeletal remains of pre-Columbian American Indians, with much less definitive findings of a similar nature in Old World skeletons [2]. Moreover, the Columbian theory gains credence in that this previously unknown disease spread like wildfire throughout Europe following the return of Columbus from the Americas and the ensuing outbreak of the first Italian War between France and Spain in 1495.

Waged in Italy (Kingdom of Naples), King Charles VIII's mercenary French troops from across Europe engaged in orgies of rape and pillage in Naples and other cities during the Italian War, contracting this new and terrible disease. Following their (and female camp followers) post-war return to their home countries, a massive epidemic of syphilis—frequently slandered as the "French Pox"—began spreading throughout Europe [2]. According to the post-Columbus school of thought, Spaniards who participated in the war and had accompanied Columbus to the Americas likely infected the local population of Naples with a critical number of seed cases.

Of interest, the name *syphilis* was coined in 1530 by the Italian physician and poet Girolamo Fracastoro, making metaphoric reference to the mythical Greek shepherd, Syphilus, who was cursed by the god Apollo with a dreadful disease [2].

****

Epidemics of syphilis have occurred repeatedly throughout history, frequently accompanying wars. The American Civil War is a prime example. Young men, filled to the brim with testosterone, unencumbered by parental or church supervision, emboldened by alcohol, and facing deadly conflict, were susceptible to the temptations of the fairer sex (Fig. 5.1).

Houses of prostitution adorned every major city during the Civil War era and female "camp followers" provided sexual services to soldiers wherever they traveled. Military records indicate that over 100,000 Union soldiers were court-martialed for sexual misconduct during the war and a concluding report by the Surgeon General at the end of the war listed 183,000 cases of venereal disease in the Union

Fig. 5.1 Civil war sexual temptation cartoon. (Picture Source: www. artsci.case.edu/dittrick. Dittrick Medical History Center)

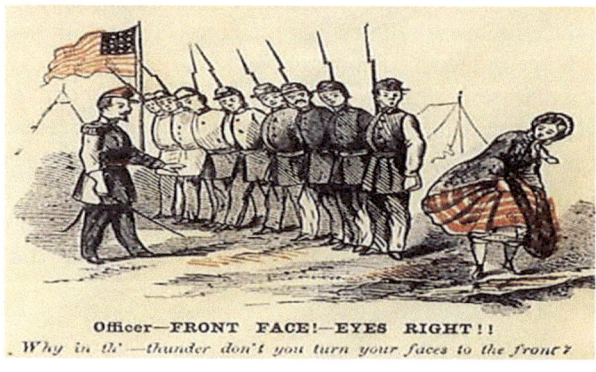

Officer—FRONT FACE!—EYES RIGHT!!
Why in th'—thunder don't you turn your faces to the front ?

Fig. 5.2 "You can't beat the Axis if you get VD". WWII poster warning about the spread of venereal diseases. (Picture Source: https://www.nlm.nih.gov. National Library of Medicine)

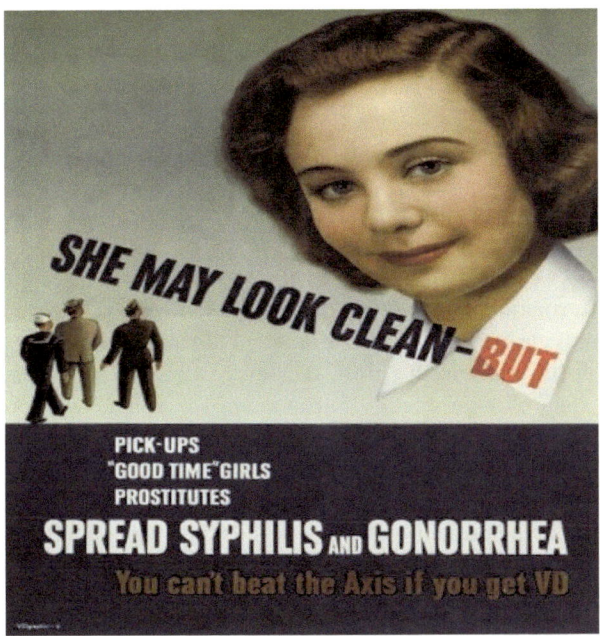

Army [3]. Likely, many cases went unreported or undetected and the numbers within the Confederate Army are undocumented—but presumptively of similar magnitude.

Among White Union troops, records indicate over 73,000 were treated for syphilis and 109,000 for gonorrhea [3]. Black soldiers accounted for many fewer cases, being less in overall number and, perhaps, less inclined to interact with White prostitutes due to social stigmas. Condoms were available to soldiers through mail order or other means but, clearly, were not used by everyone or, perhaps, not during every encounter. Repeated usage may have limited their effectiveness, as well.

To counteract the epidemic of venereal disease, the military opened licensed houses of prostitution in several cities. Women of "vile character" were excluded. Periodic medical exams of the prostitutes were required and those afflicted were hospitalized and treated. The program met with some success, the Surgeon General reporting, "*while it does not encourage vice it prevents to a considerable extent its worst consequences*" [3]. Soldiers, of course, took the scourge of venereal disease home with them, furthering the epidemic.

Similar spikes of venereal disease occurred among soldiers in WWI and WWII, despite extensive efforts in sex education, ubiquitous propaganda posters warning of the dangers of unprotected sexual encounters and the distribution of condoms (Fig. 5.2). The cost to the Army in lost time from duty and diversion of medical resources was enormous, as well as a source of political and social tension between American forces and their Allied host nations [4, 5].

****

First identified by German zoologist Fritz Schaudinn (1871–1906) and dermatologist Eric Hoffmann (1868–1959) in 1905 [6], the cause of syphilis is now known to be a corkscrew-shaped bacterium within the *Treponema* group of spirochetes called *Treponema pallidum*. The bacterium is generally transmitted from person to person through sexual intercourse, but may also be transmitted from mother to baby during pregnancy or at birth, resulting in congenital syphilis. Humans are the only known natural reservoir for the *pallidum* subspecies, which has an uncanny ability to evade the immune system.

Untreated, the disease is nasty. The first stage of syphilis is characterized by the formation of a painless ulcerative chancre on the penis (or tongue) or within the vagina or anus. Without treatment the infection may appear to resolve, only to transform into a rash (Fig. 5.3), fever, sore throat, headache, or hair loss (secondary stage), or go directly into a latent stage. The asymptomatic latent stage may last several years, leading to the false assumption of a cure. In the final (tertiary) stage, affecting 20–30% of infected patients, the central nervous system, eyes, brain or heart may be attacked, frequently resulting in death [7].

In the pre-antibiotic era, syphilis was treated with mercury, bismuth, arsenic, and other heavy metal injections (Fig. 5.4), salves, and suffumigations (sweat baths). The intrinsic toxicity of these substances is self-evident and most of the early preparations and treatment protocols are now recognized as non-curative. Therapeutic regimens often lasted for years, giving rise to the euphemism, "A night with Venus, and a lifetime with mercury" [8, 9].

The arsenical arsphenamine (marketed in 1910 as *Salvarsan*) achieved some success in treating syphilis, and in combination with small doses of bismuth or mercury became the standard of treatment until the introduction of penicillin in the 1940s [9, 10].

In 1917 an Australian physician Julius Wagner-Jauregg (1857–1940) introduced a completely different and unique treatment concept. He observed that the symptoms of tertiary neurosyphilis diminished after febrile illnesses. His therapeutic modality was to infect patients with malaria parasites, rationalizing that the treatment of malaria was simpler and more successful than treating syphilis [11]. The concept awarded him a Nobel Prize in 1927 but never received widespread

Fig. 5.3 Secondary syphilis rash. (Picture Source: https://www.cdc. gov. CDC)

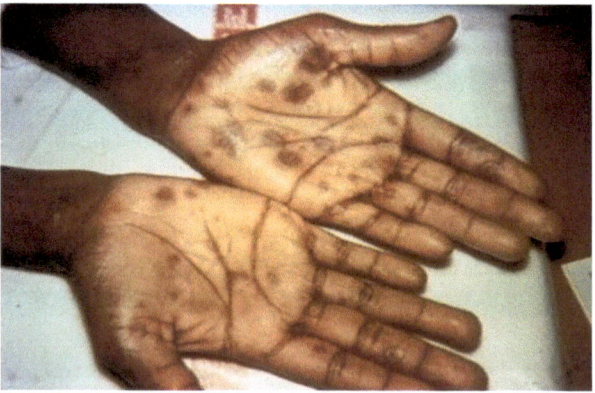

Fig. 5.4 Heavy metal injection granulomas in gluteal muscles: a common pre-antibiotic treatment for syphilis. (Picture Source: Author's collection)

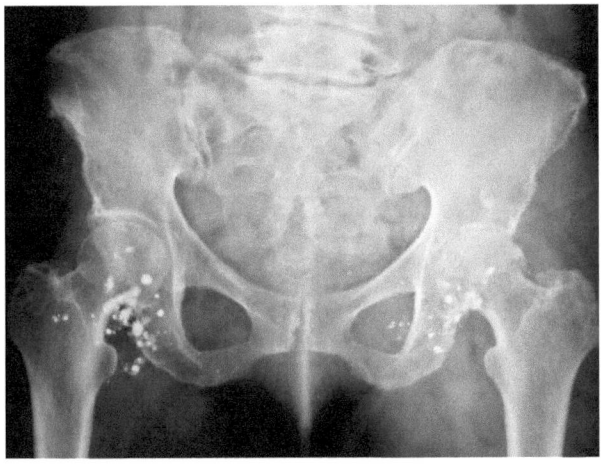

acceptance. Suffice it to say, when penicillin became available in the 1940s, all previous treatment modalities for syphilis became obsolete.

One of the most disturbing scourges in the history of U.S. medicine is the Tuskegee syphilis experiment [12] which began in 1932—at a time when there was no known curative treatment for syphilis. With a bogus promise of free medical care, 600 African American men in Macon County, Alabama, with known syphilis—often referred to as "bad blood" among the African American community—were enrolled in the project.

To track the disease's natural progression, researchers allowed the disease to progress relentlessly in the study participants, even after penicillin became available in the mid-1940s and was known to be curative. Some men died, others went blind or insane or experienced other related health problems.

Congressional hearings on the Tuskegee experiment were held in 1973. Ultimately, the study's surviving participants and heirs of the deceased received a $10 million out-of-court settlement. Importantly, new guidelines were also imposed to protect human test subjects in subsequent government-funded research projects.

****

In addition to clinical evaluation, the laboratory diagnosis of syphilis [13] may involve dark-field microscopy of skin lesions (if present), but most often involves serological screening with a non-treponemal specific antigen test (e.g., VDRL, RPR) and, if positive, confirmation with a treponemal-specific test (e.g., FTA, EIA). In some instances, the non-specific tests may be skipped (or used in reversed sequencing) if the diagnosis seems clear-cut based on the patient's history or clinical examination.

A single injection of long-acting benzathine penicillin G is generally curative for primary, secondary, and early stages of late syphilis. Three doses at weekly intervals are recommended for late latent syphilis or latent syphilis of unknown duration. Alternative antibiotics are also effective for those with penicillin allergies. Of note,

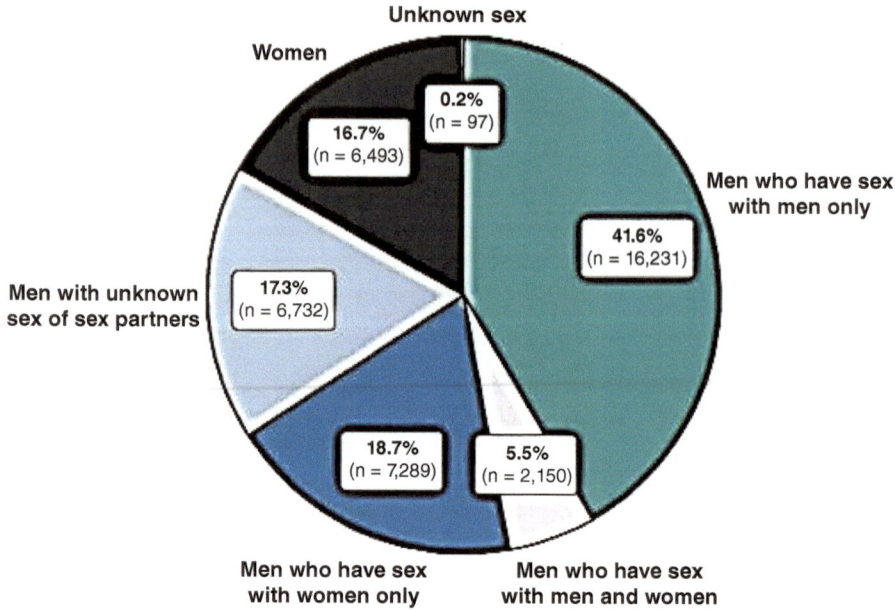

Fig. 5.5 Distribution of primary and secondary syphilis cases in the USA, 2019. (Picture Source: https://www.cdc.gov. CDC)

antibiotic treatment does not reverse ancillary organ or tissue damage that may have been done by untreated syphilis [14].

In 2019, 129,813 cases of syphilis were reported in the USA according to the CDC. Among those were 38,992 cases of the more infectious primary and secondary stages, distributed according to the type of sexual partner, as shown below (Fig. 5.5) [15].

Of alarming concern is the current rise in newborn syphilis cases (congenital syphilis) in the USA, resulting from expectant mothers not receiving appropriate testing and treatment during pregnancy [16]. Syphilis during pregnancy can cause miscarriage, stillbirth, infant death, and a plethora of lifelong medical problems in affected children [17].

According to the CDC, more than 3700 babies were born with syphilis in 2022, representing a ten-fold rise in cases since 2012 [16]. The cause of this increase is thought to be multifactorial, including an overall increase in syphilis infections among women of childbearing age, coupled with social, racial, and economic barriers, most notably within minority ethnic groups, to high-quality prenatal care [16].

Gonorrhea (*"The Clap," "The Drip"*)

Gonorrhea is a sexually transmitted disease (STD) caused by the *Neisseria gonorrhoeae* bacterium, first identified as the infecting organism by Albert L. S. Neisser (1855–1916) in 1879 [18]. An ancient disease dating back to the beginnings of written history [19], gonorrhea remains one of the most commonly occurring STDs in the USA, with an estimated 1.6 million cases occurring in 2018, according to the CDC [20].

N. Gonorrhoeae is transferred from one person to another through vaginal, oral, and anal sex, infecting the mucous membranes of the reproductive tract, urethra, throat or rectum, depending on the site of sexual interaction. Ejaculation is not necessary for disease transmission. A newborn may become infected during childbirth and those persons with prior infections which were curatively treated may become reinfected following a subsequent exposure [20].

Both men and women with active infections can remain asymptomatic, making accurate estimates of disease incidence difficult and distinct from reported case statistics. Women with symptomatic infections may note dysuria (pain on urination), vaginal discharge, spot bleeding between menstrual periods, pain in the pelvic area and dyspareunia (pain with intercourse). Men with symptomatic infections commonly experience urethritis, purulent discharge from the penis, and testicular pain and/or swelling. A sore throat or difficulty swallowing may follow oral sex, and itching, discharge or pain when defecating may follow anal intercourse [20, 21].

If untreated, women may develop pelvic inflammatory disease (PID) and men epididymitis, both of which can lead to infertility. Spread of the infecting organism to the bloodstream may result in septic arthritis or tenosynovitis, liver inflammation, heart valve or brain damage and may be life threatening. An infant born to a mother with a gonococcal cervical infection may develop infective conjunctivitis which can spread to the cornea and cause permanent vision damage. Although now rare, newborn gonococcal conjunctivitis was once a major cause of blindness in the USA [20–22].

As there is no effective vaccine for gonorrhea, avoidance of the disease is best achieved by abstinence from sexual relations, monogamous sex with a non-infected individual, or correct and unwavering use of a condom. The diagnosis of gonococcal infection is based on clinical history and physical examination, but a microbiologic diagnosis is required due to the similar presentation of other STDs. In general, nucleic acid amplification testing (NAAT) is the test of choice for the initial microbiologic diagnosis of *N. gonorrhoeae* infection, although culture of endocervical or urethral swabs remains an important diagnostic tool when antibiotic resistance is suspected [20, 23].

Light microscopy histopathology of cervical or urethral swabs in a patient infected with gonorrhea typically shows gram-negative intracellular (within white cells) diplococcus bacteria, as shown in the low-resolution photomicrograph below (Fig. 5.6).

If infected, treatment consists of antibiotics, with a single 500mg intramuscular dose of ceftriaxone being the current recommendation [20, 21]. Persistent symptoms following antibiotic administration suggest a drug-resistant strain which generally necessitates organism culture to determine drug sensitivity and supplemental or alternative antibiotic administration.

****

Fig. 5.6 Photomicrograph
of a gonococcal smear.
CDC/Joe Millar. (Picture
Source: https://en.
wikipedia.org. CDC:
Public Health Image
Library)

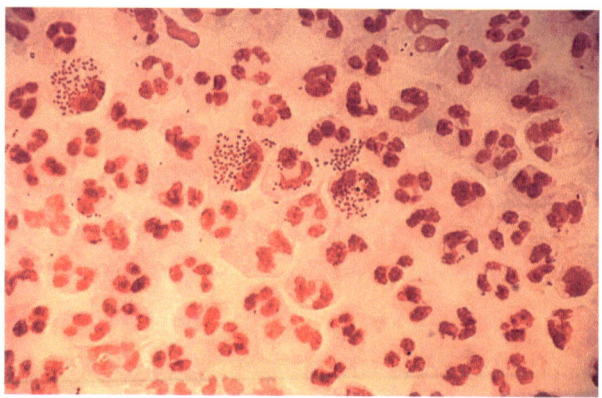

Gonorrhea derives its name from the Greek, meaning "the flow of seed" (gono: seed, rhea: flow). The term is credited to the preeminent Greek physician Galen (131–200 CE), who apparently mistook the purulent exudate emanating from the penis as an unwanted flow of semen [19, 24]. Less clear is the origin of the common moniker, "The Clap." Among other possibilities, the nickname is thought to be derived from the ancient practice of clapping the sides of the infected penis to extrude pus. French brothels were known as "Les Clapiers"—often attributed to the origin of infections—representing another possibility. The descriptive "Drip" moniker is somewhat self-evident in its origin, as a purulent exudate emanating from the penis or vagina is a common sign of gonococcal infections [24, 25].

Prior to the introduction of penicillin in the 1940s, gonorrhea was treated with a variety of caustic urethral/vaginal irrigates, including a variety of mercury, potassium, and silver compounds. In the early twentieth century heat therapy was advocated and thought to be curative. Patients were placed in a "fever cabinet" encasing the body (but not the head) and exposed to temperatures around 41 °C (106 °F) for a number of hours over several sequential days, with some success. Sulfonamide antibiotics became available in 1937 and were initially effective in curing gonorrhea, but bacterial resistance rapidly ensued. In the early 1940s penicillin became the mainstay of treatment, followed by multiple other alternative antibiotics as resistant strains developed [24].

Universally, wars have brought about a dramatic surge in STD cases within the military, as an ethos of drinking, gambling, and sexual debauchery has long been embraced by many combatants facing the horrors of war, across all time and cultures. As noted in the previous section on syphilis, a concluding report by the Surgeon General of the USA at the end of the Civil War listed 183,000 cases of venereal disease in the Union Army, with records indicating over 73,000 White troops were treated for syphilis and 109,000 for gonorrhea [26, 27].

During World War I, the U.S. Army lost 6,804,818 duty days and discharged more than 10,000 men because of STDs, only surpassed in sick time by those afflicted by the influenza pandemic of 1918–1919 [27, 28]. A similar spike of venereal disease occurred among soldiers in WWII, prompting extensive efforts in sex

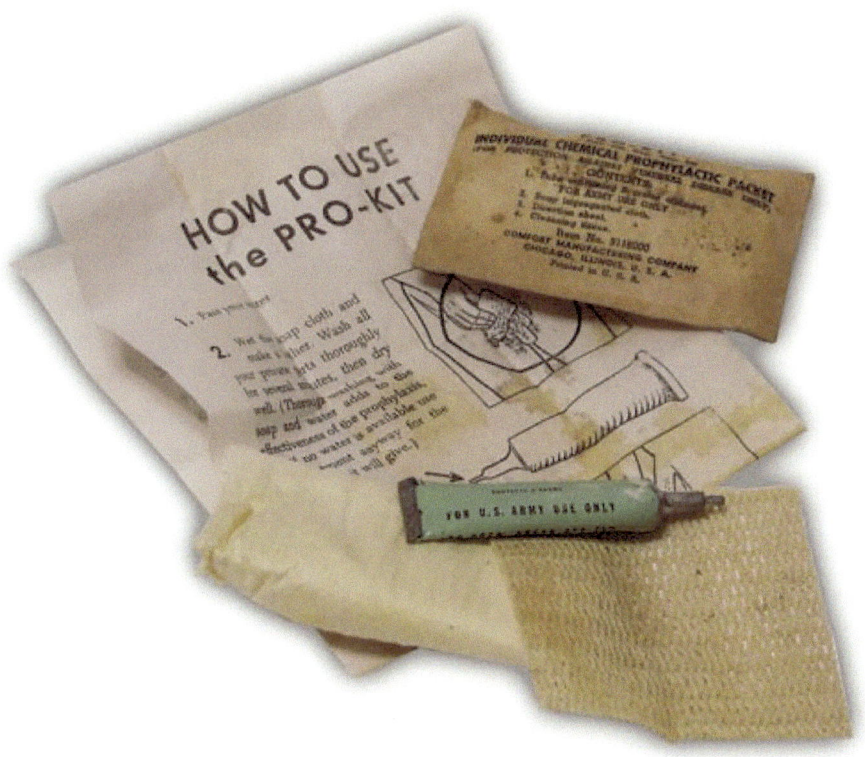

Fig. 5.7 The "individual prophylactic packet" administered to soldiers in WWII. Item # 9118000. (Picture Source: https://www.med-dept.com. WW2 US Medical Research Center)

education, ubiquitous posters warning of the dangers of unprotected sex [29], and the distribution of condoms and *Individual Chemical Prophylactic Packets* (Fig. 5.7), containing cleansing tissues and a tube of ointment (30% mercury chloride mineral and 15% Sulfathiazole) for urethral injection to be used immediately after a sexual encounter [30].

In both world wars the cost to the U.S. Army in lost time from service and the diversion of medical resources to treat STDs was enormous. Prior to the introduction of penicillin, treating syphilis with a protracted series of heavy metal injections was a 6-month ordeal. A case of gonorrhea often necessitated a hospital stay of 30 days. After penicillin introduction in mid-1944, the length of military hospital stays decreased dramatically and, in many cases, treatment no longer required hospitalization or significantly impacted operational readiness [27, 28, 30].

****

According to the CDC, the reported incidence of gonorrhea infections in the USA has increased since 2009 (Fig. 5.8) and rates among men have increased

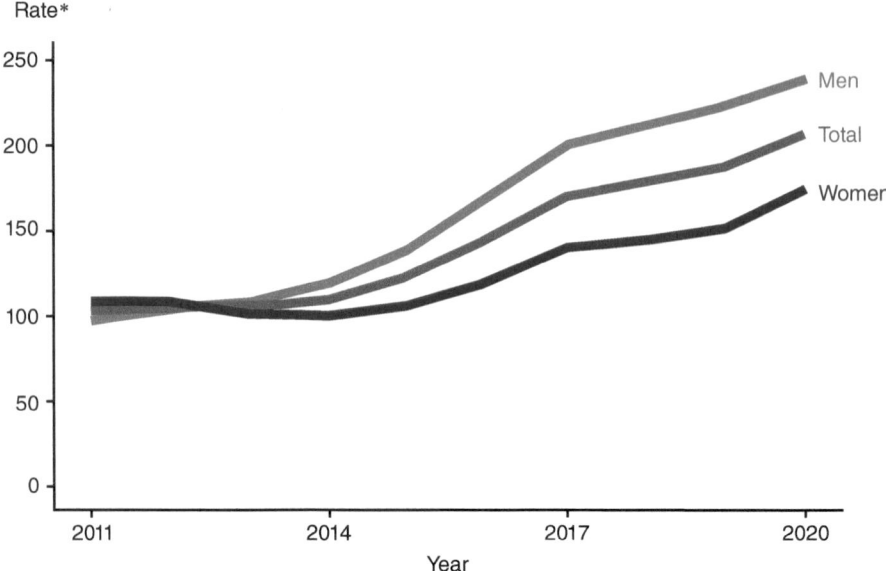

Fig. 5.8 Number of reported gonorrhea cases per 100,000 persons in the USA (2011–2020). (Picture Source: https://www.cdc.gov/std/statistics/2020. CDC)

disproportionately to women, perhaps reflecting an increase in the prevalence of sex between men [20]. Antibiotic resistance remains a concern, with half of the gonococcal isolates since 2020 showing some antibiotic resistance, although resistance to ceftriaxone (the current primary treatment for gonorrhea) remains rare [20].

References

Syphilis

1. Porter R. The greatest benefit to mankind: a medical history of humanity. New York: W.W. Norton & Company, Inc.; 1998.
2. Tampa M, Sarbu I, Matel C, et al. Brief history of syphilis. J Med Life. 2014;7(1):4–10. https://www.ncbi.nlm.nih.gov.
3. Dittrick Medical History Center. The Civil War: sex and soldiers. Cleveland: Case Western Reserve University; 2022. https://artsci.case.edu/dittrick.
4. Speaker SL. "Fit to fight": home front army doctors and VD during WWI. Circulating Now: from the historical collection of the National Library of Medicine. 2018. https://circulating-now.nlm.nih.gov.
5. WW2 US Medical Research Centre. Venereal disease and treatment during WW2. WW2 US Medical Research Centre; 2007. https://www.med-dept.com.
6. Linda Hall Library. Fritz Schaudinn. Linda Hall Library; 2022. https://www.lindahall.org.
7. CDC. Syphilis—CDC detailed fact sheet. Centers for Disease Control and Prevention; 2022. https://www.cdc.gov.

8. Junichi T, Shaw JA. Heavy metal injection granulomas: a source of diagnostic confusion. J Bone Joint Surg. 2002;84(5):800–3. https://pubmed.ncbi.nlm.nih.gov.

9. Frith J. Syphilis—its early history and treatment until penicillin and the debate on its origin. J Mil Vet Hist. 2021;20(4):49–58. https://jmvh.org.

10. Williams KJ. The introduction of 'chemotherapy' using arsphenamine—the first magic bullet. J R Soc Med. 2009;102(8):343–8. https://www.ncbi.nlm.nih.gov.

11. Vanhave JP. Treatment of syphilis with malaria or heat. Ned Tijdschr Geneeskd. 2016;160:A9852. https://pubmed.ncbi.nlm.nih.gov.

12. Nix E. Tuskegee experiment: the infamous syphilis study. History. 2020. https://www.history.com.

13. IDPH. Increasing early syphilis cases in Illinois—syphilis laboratory tests. Springfield: Illinois Department of Public Health; 2022. https://www.dph.illinois.gov.

14. CDC. Syphilis treatment and care. Centers for Disease Control and Prevention; 2022. https://www.cdc.gov.

15. CDC. National overview—sexually transmitted disease surveillance. Centers for Disease Control and Prevention; 2019. https://www.cdc.gov.

16. CDC. U.S. syphilis cases in newborns continue to increase: a 10-times increase over a decade. Centers for Disease Control and Prevention; 2023. https://www.cdc.gov.

17. Tesini BL. Congenital syphilis. Merck Manual: professional version. 2022. https://www.merckmanuals.com.

Gonorrhea

18. Ligon BL. Albert Ludwig Sigesmund Neisser: discoverer of the cause of gonorrhea. Semin Pediatr Infect Dis. 2005;16(4):336–41. https://pubmed.ncbi.nlm.nih.gov.

19. Vicentini CB, Manfredini S, Maritati M, et al. Gonorrhea, a current disease with ancient roots: from the remedies of the past to future perspectives. Infez Med. 2019;27(2):212–21. https://pubmed.ncbi.nlm.nih.gov.

20. CDC. Gonorrhea—CDC detailed fact sheet. Centers for Disease Control and Prevention; 2022. https://www.cdc.gov.

21. Cleveland Clinic. Gonorrhea: causes, symptoms, treatment and prevention. Cleveland: Cleveland Clinic; 2022. https://my.clevelandclinic.org.

22. Jin J. Prevention of gonococcal eye infection in newborns. JAMA. 2019;321(4):414. https://jamanetwork.com.

23. Meyer T, Buder S. The laboratory diagnosis of *Neisseria gonorrhoeae*: current testing and future demands. Pathogens. 2020;9(2):91. https://www.ncbi.nlm.nih.gov.

24. Jose PP, Vivekanandan V, Sobhanakumari K. Gonorrhea: historical outlook. J Skin Sex Transm Dis. 2020;2(2):110. https://jstd.org.

25. Wooldridge A. Why is gonorrhea called the clap? K Health; 2022. https://khealth.com.

26. Murphy LR. The enemy among us: venereal disease among union soldiers in the far west. Civil War Hist. 1985;31(3):257–69. https://muse.jhu.edu.

27. Rasnake MS, Conger NG, McAllister CK, et al. History of U.S. military contributions to the study of sexually transmitted diseases. Mil Med. 2005;170(4):61–5. https://www.afids.org.

28. Speaker SL. "Fit to fight": home front army doctors and VD during WW I. Circulating Now. National Library of Medicine; 2018. https://circulatingnow.nlm.nih.gov.

29. Gettleman E, Murrmann M. The enemy in your pants: the military's decades-long war against STDs. Mother Jones. 2010. https://www.motherjones.com.

30. WW2 US Medical Research Center. Venereal disease and treatment during WW2. WW2 US Medical Research Center; 2007. https://med-dept.com.

Chapter 6
Substance Use Disorders

Abstract Substance use disorders are self-inflicted indulgences, often resulting in addictions. Alcohol and opioid use and abuse have plagued Americans throughout history, notably during the nineteenth century, during periods of war, and during recent years referrable to heroin, prescription drug, and synthetic opioid (fentanyl) abuse. Dramatic periods of history, including the Prohibition era, are an integral part of the American experience referable to alcohol use disorder.

The substance use disorders discussed in this chapter, along with their historical names and monikers, are: Alcohol Use Disorder (*Barrel Fever*) and Opioid Use Disorder (*Laudanum Euphoria, Soldier's Disease*).

Alcohol Use Disorder (*Barrel Fever*)

Alcoholic beverages have been brewed by humans since the dawn of time and their use and abuse have played a prominent role in American history from its inception to the present time. In the period before the American Revolution, colonialists drank heavily as part of their daily routines and alcohol played a prominent role as a "social lubricant" during personal gatherings and community events. Native Americans were plied with alcohol as a means of weakening their resistance to unreasonable demands for land, resources, furs, and women (Fig. 6.1). Revenue for financially strapped colonial governments relied heavily on alcohol taxes [1–3].

In the pre-Revolution period, drunkenness was regarded as a moral weakness and those imbibing to excess were pilloried from the pulpit and locked in stocks for public shaming. Following the Revolution, sentiment regarding alcohol abuse began to change. The drunkard was no longer regarded as lacking moral fortitude but an unwitting victim of an addictive and poisonous substance—creating the foundational voice for the temperance societies of the 1800s and 1900s [1, 2].

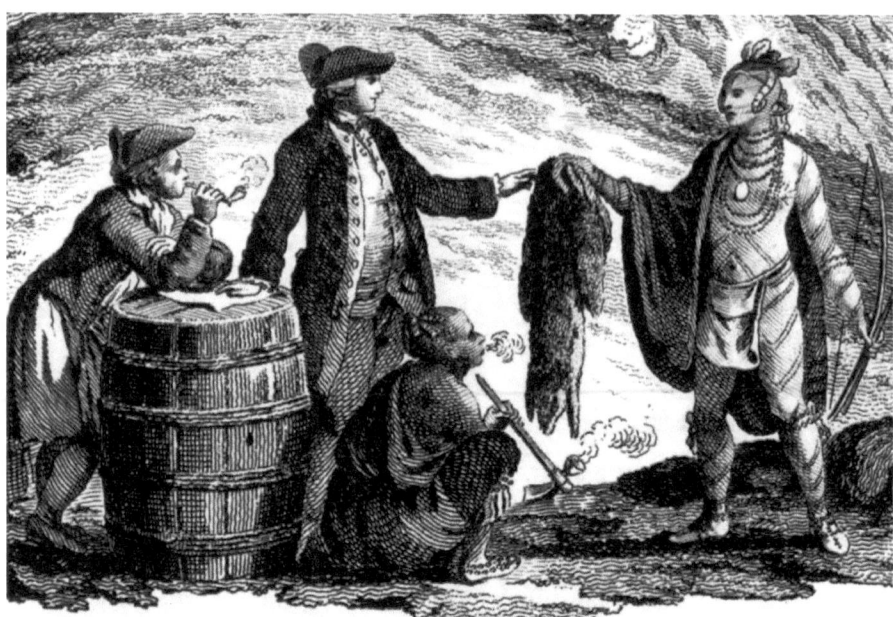

Fig. 6.1 European fur traders bargaining with a barrel of rum. From William Faden: "A Map of the Inhabited Part of Canada from the French Surveys; with the Frontiers of New York and New England," 1777. (Picture Source: https://en.wikipedia.org. Library and Archives Canada)

Chronic alcohol abuse was rampant within the USA throughout the nineteenth century, with estimates suggesting that Americans over 15 years of age consumed nearly three times as much alcohol in 1830 as they do today [4]. Alcohol-related spousal abuse, family neglect, and chronic unemployment were scourges on society. Women and children, who were dependent on their husbands' and fathers' financial support, often suffered physical and emotional abuse and economic uncertainty (Fig. 6.2). Employers had to deal with intoxicated workers and an unreliable labor force on a frequent basis [4, 5].

In response, the temperance movement took hold in a pervasive fashion during the 1830s and 1840s, spearheaded mostly by women and Protestant religious groups (Fig. 6.3). Initially, drinkers were urged to resist the temptation of alcohol and imbibe only in moderation. As the movement gained momentum, temperance groups began to demand that local, state, and national governments ban alcohol entirely. Bowing to public sentiment, states started to pass prohibition laws in the 1850s, first initiated by the state of Maine ("Maine Laws") on June 2, 1851 [4–6].

The Civil War dealt the temperance movement a crippling—albeit temporary—blow. With the compelling issues of slavery, states' rights, and war-related matters on the minds of most people, concerns over alcohol abuse seemed of secondary importance and the movement was back-peddled into relative obscurity. Of equal impediment was the fact that both the North and the South financed the war in large part by taxing breweries and distilleries, making Prohibition fiscally untenable. For

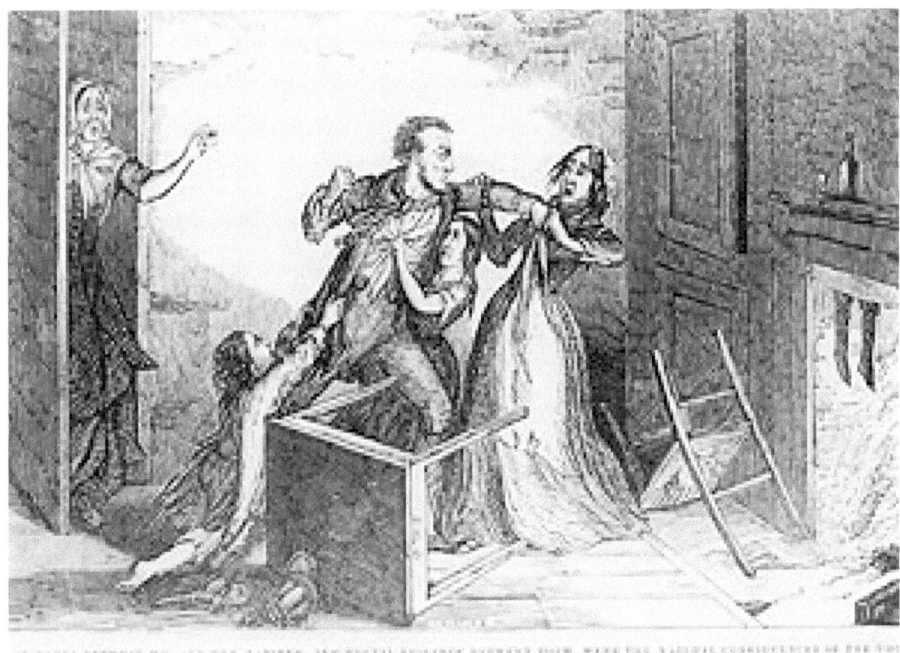

Fig. 6.2 Temperance illustration of a drunkard husband abusing his wife. From: The Bottle, 1847. (Picture Source: https://www.pbs.org. Library of Congress)

the most part, Prohibition laws in effect at the beginning of the war were all repealed by the end of the war [6].

That said, temperance sentiment never disappeared during the war years and sprang back with a vengeance in the 1870s. With women's groups, such as the Woman's Christian Temperance Union (WCTU), and the all-male, politically astute, Anti-Saloon League (ASL) championing the movement, American citizens of all persuasions began to lend support to the temperance crusade. Anti-German sentiment in the throes of WWI linked German beer to treason in the minds of some people and may have added impetus to the temperance movement as well [5, 6].

Of importance, the 16th Amendment to the U.S. Constitution (Feb. 3, 1913) established Congress's right to impose a federal income tax, freeing the Federal Government from dependence on alcohol-related taxes as its principal source of revenue, making prohibition fiscally tenable.

Ultimately, under the combination of influences noted above, the temperance movement triumphed with the passage of the 18th Amendment to the Constitution by Congress on December 18, 1917. Ratified by the requisite three-fourths of the states on January 16, 1919, and passed into law a year later, the amendment declared that the production, transport, and sale of intoxicating liquors (but not consumption) was illegal. Popularly known as the "Volstead Act," the *National Prohibition Act*

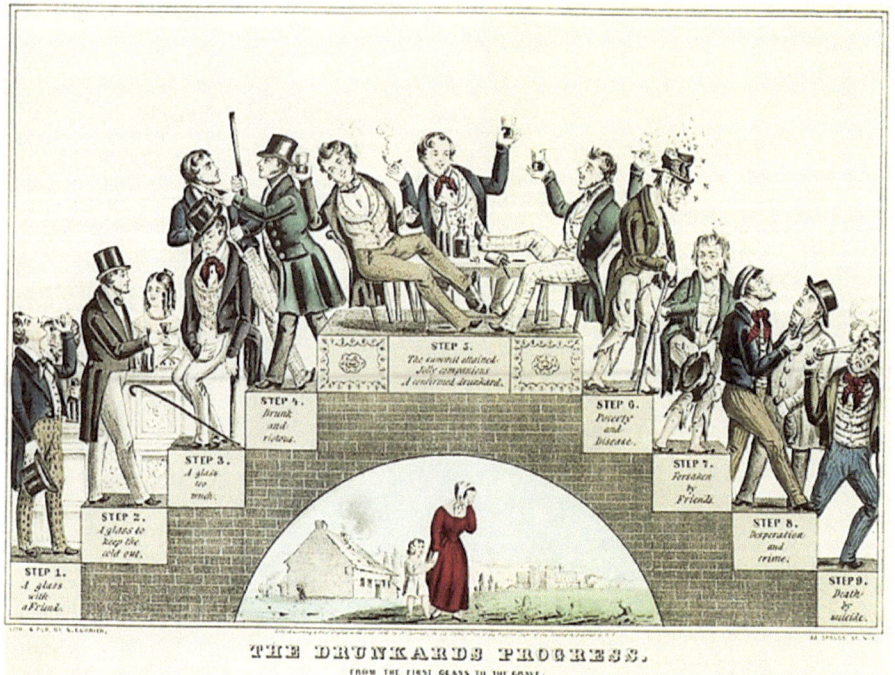

Fig. 6.3 Temperance poster depicting the Drunkards Progress, Circa 1846. (1) A glass with a friend, (2) A glass to keep the cold out, (3) A glass too much, (4) Drunk and riotous, (5) A confirmed drunkard, (6) Poverty and disease, (7) Forsaken by friends, (8) Desperation and crime, (9) Death by suicide. N. Currier (firm). (Picture Source: https://www.loc.gov. Library of Congress)

was subsequently enacted to provide the government with the means of enforcing the Prohibition Amendment.

Be that as it may, victory was short-lived for the temperance movement. In overt defiance of the 18th Amendment, many Americans began brewing alcoholic beverages at home and imbibed illegally acquired spirits with little regard for the law. Organized crime (bootleggers) imported and distributed beer and liquor virtually unabated. Police enforced Prohibition laws lackadaisically and almost every saloon that was shuttered during the Prohibition Era was replaced by a bevy of "speakeasies."

On December 5, 1933, the 21st Amendment was ratified, repealing the 18th Amendment. After 13 years of Prohibition (and in the midst of the Great Depression), Congress and a majority of American citizens had come to the realization that the 18th Amendment had caused more problems than it solved. The manufacture, sale, and transport of alcohol became legal once again [4–6].

****

Alcohol use disorder (AUD), as defined by the National Institute on Alcohol Abuse and Alcoholism [7], is a medical condition:

> Characterized by an impaired ability to stop or control alcohol use despite adverse social, occupational, or health consequences. It encompasses the conditions that some people refer to as alcohol abuse, alcohol dependence, alcohol addiction, and the colloquial term, alcoholism.

The 2021 National Survey on Drug Use and Health (NSDUH) identified 29.5 million people ages 12 and older (10.6% in this age group) with AUD within the USA [8]. Among U.S. citizens, Native Americans may be particularly susceptible to AUD, according to American Addiction Centers [9], attributed to multiple factors, including historical trauma, lack of ready access to health care, lower educational attainment, poverty, unemployment, violence, and loss of cultural connection, among others. WHO statistics indicate that approximately 3 million deaths (5.3% of all deaths) occur each year worldwide as a result of alcohol abuse, with alcohol accounting for 13.5% of deaths in people aged 20–39 years of age [10].

Alcohol use disorder may include periods of intoxication and periods of symptomatic alcohol withdrawal. An intoxicated individual typically displays physical, mental, and behavioral changes that are markedly deviant from normalcy, while excessively high blood alcohol levels can lead to coma, brain damage, and death. Symptomatic alcohol withdrawal results from abrupt cessation of alcohol consumption in an individual with a history of heavy and prolonged use. Referred to as *delirium tremens* (DTs) within the medical community and "barrel fever" in slang terminology, acute withdrawal may result in fever, tremors, hallucinations, severe agitation, seizures, and death [11, 12].

Treatment approaches for AUD vary from individual to individual, but may include medication (naltrexone, acamprosate, and disulfiram), behavioral modification therapy, and mutual-support groups. Many people do recover successfully from AUD, but a relapse of drinking behavior is common [7].

Opioid Use Disorder (*Laudanum Euphoria, Soldier's Disease*)

Opioid use and abuse remain at epidemic levels in the USA at this time, as evidenced by almost daily headline news. Recent data suggests that three million persons in the USA and 16 million persons worldwide have been afflicted by opioid use disorder (OUD) at some point during their lives [13]. In 2021 more than 106,000 persons died in America from drug overdoses according to the National Institute on Drug Abuse (Fig. 6.4) [14].

CDC data indicates that the current synthetic opioid overdose death wave—principally involving illicitly manufactured fentanyl—began in 2013 and was preceded by a wave of heroin overdoses starting in 2010 and a prescription opioid overdose

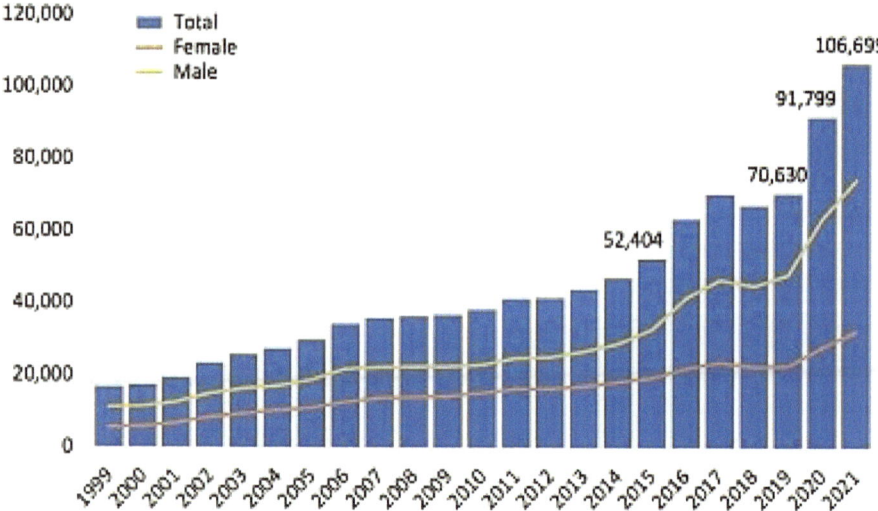

Fig. 6.4 Drug-involved overdose deaths in the USA (1999–2021). (Picture Source: https://nida.nih.gov. NIH: National Institute on Drug Abuse)

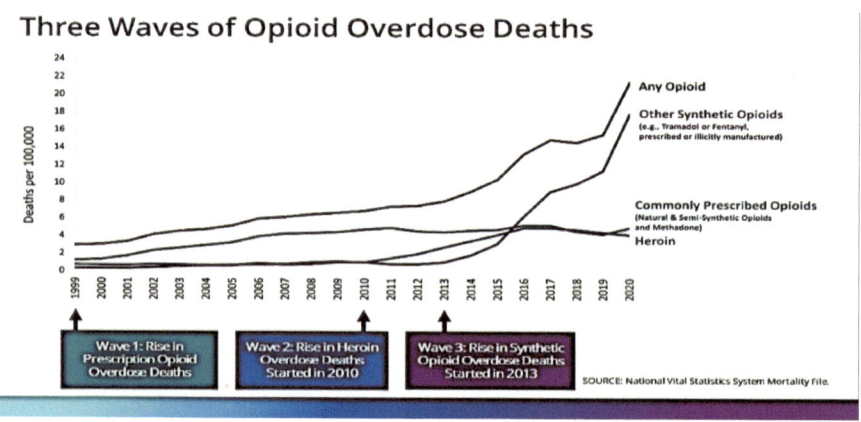

Fig. 6.5 Prescription opioid, heroin, and synthetic opioid. Death Waves in the USA (1999–2020). (Picture Source: https://www.cdc.gov. CDC)

wave (oxycodone and hydrocodone) starting around 1999 [15]. From 1999 to 2020 more than 564,000 persons died in the USA from opioid overdose, both prescription and illicit [15].

More recently, opioid overdose deaths within the USA increased by 38% in the interval between 2019 and 2020 (Fig. 6.5), with synthetic opioid-involved deaths predominating with a rate increase of 56% [15].

****

Opium use dates back thousands of years, but America's first true opioid crisis dates to the Civil War and its immediate aftermath [16–18]. Opium pills, morphine injections, and laudanum—a tincture of alcohol and opium—were widely used during the war to treat pain and control diarrhea and coughs (Fig. 6.6). Over-prescribing by military physicians and prolonged usage, principally among maimed soldiers and those suffering from dysentery, led to life-long addiction in many instances. An estimated 400,000 soldiers returned home addicted to morphine; a condition often referred to as "Soldiers Disease" [19].

Within the civilian population, laudanum and other similar opioid-containing "patent medicines" could be purchased virtually anywhere—grocery stores, barber shops, tobacconists, and pharmacies, among many other places—at prices readily affordable to most people. As noted previously, they were unscrupulously marketed as cures for virtually every human ailment, including depression, rheumatism, digestive ailments, melancholy, gout, and "women's problems."

With unfortunate parallels to the current opioid crisis, laudanum addiction became a scourge of the nineteenth century. Medicinal excuses and feigned illnesses were proffered by persons across all levels of society to cover for their underlying psychological and physical dependency on laudanum or similar opioid-containing compounds [20–22].

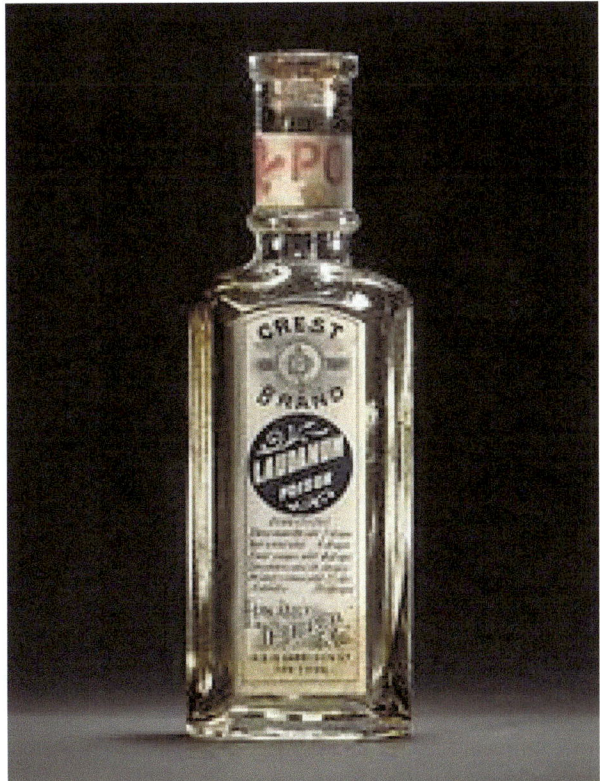

Fig. 6.6 Laudanum: Edward D. Depew & Co. Circa 1880. (Picture Source: https://www.nlm.nih.gov. Nat. Museum of American History)

Thought to be responsible for many infant deaths from overdose and/or opiate withdrawal, one of the most ill-reputed patent medicines was "Mrs. Winslow's Soothing Syrup." Laced with morphine and alcohol, the syrup was introduced in 1849 and aggressively marketed for decades to parents of fussy children, particularly those undergoing teething (Fig. 6.7). The syrup and other patent medicines were called to task in 1906 when the Federal Government passed the landmark *Pure Food and Drug Act*, requiring product labels to list "addictive" and/or "dangerous" ingredients, including alcohol, morphine, opium, and cannabis [20–22].

During WW I, soldiers often used cocaine to boost energy, lessen combat fatigue, and reduce anxiety. In this regard, Burroughs Wellcome & Co. produced an army-issued drug known as "Forced March," containing cocaine and cola nut extract (Fig. 6.8). Purported to "allay hunger and prolong the power of endurance," directions for use stated that a tablet should be: *"Dissolved in the mouth every hour when undergoing continued mental strain or physical exertion"* [19].

Amphetamines were the most widely used drug during WW II. Spearheaded by the Nazis with the introduction of Pervitin (an early version of methamphetamine), U.S., British and Japanese armies also used amphetamines (Benzedrine) during the war to foster confidence, enhance energy and performance, and help troops stay awake for prolonged periods during combat [19].

The sanctioned use and administration of amphetamines (dextroamphetamine) continued during the Vietnam War, often taken in conjunction with marijuana, opium or heroin on a self-administered basis. Formal detox programs were rarely available to combatants, and soldiers frequently suffered serious withdrawal

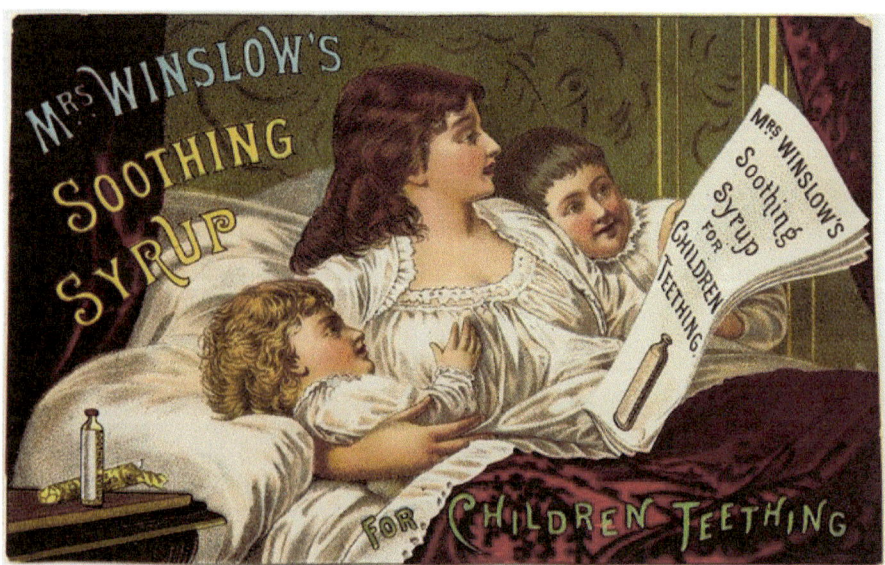

Fig. 6.7 Advertisement: Mrs. Winslow's Soothing Syrup. (Picture Source: https://www.collections.nlm.nih.gov. Nat. Library of Medicine)

Fig. 6.8 "Forced March" tablets issued in WWI. Circa 1920. (Picture Source: https://www.cocaine.org/forcedmarch.htm. Burroughs Wellcome and Co)

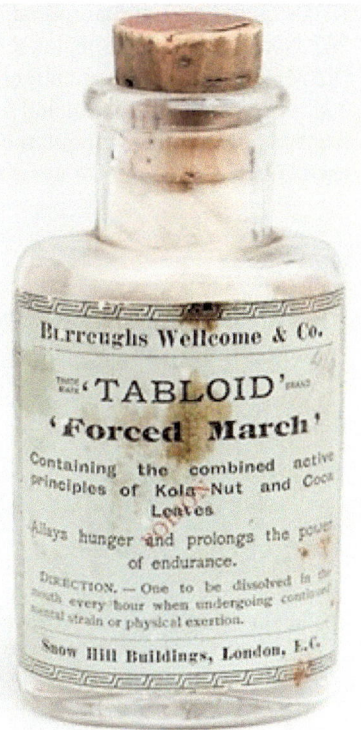

symptoms and continued addiction cravings when arriving home—often with little or no support or formal rehabilitation structure in place [19].

****

Opioids are highly addictive, inducing a feeling of intense euphoria triggered by the release of endogenously produced endorphins. Endorphins block the perception of pain and boost feelings of pleasure and a sense of well-being. With repeated opioid use, physiologic endorphin production slows, necessitating more frequent or higher doses of the drug to produce the same euphoric high, fostering addiction potential while simultaneously posing the risk of a toxic/life-threatening overdose [13, 23].

Anyone taking opioids is at risk of developing OUD, characterized by the compulsive use and irresistible craving for the drug, despite harmful social and personal consequences. Problematically, cessation of an opioid can lead to intensely unpleasant withdrawal symptoms, encouraging the continued use of the drug. Although rarely life-threatening, withdrawal symptoms may include sweating, chills, nausea, vomiting, agitation, anxiety, muscle pain, abdominal cramping, insomnia, and tachycardia, among others [13, 23].

Acute opioid overdose can be safely treated with naloxone, which is a competitive opioid receptor antagonist [24]. In conjunction with behavioral counseling and supervised medical care, effective drug regimens are available for the treatment of

AUD, including buprenorphine, methadone, and extended-release naltrexone [25, 26]. According to the Substance Abuse and Mental Health Services Administration (SAMHSA), these medications "operate to normalize brain chemistry, block euphoric effects of alcohol and opioids, relieve physiological cravings, and normalize body functions without the negative and euphoric effects of the substance used" [26].

> **N.B.**
> The reader might enjoy Barbara Hodgson's book: *In the Arms of Morpheus: The Tragic History of Morphine, Laudanum and Patent Medicines* (Firefly Books, Richmond Hill, ON Canada, 2001).

References

Alcohol Use Disorder

1. Editorial Staff River Oaks Treatment Center. The history of alcohol in America. River Oaks Treatment Center; 2023. https://riveroakstreatment.com.
2. Gerstein OS. Drinking in America. In: Alcohol in America: taking action to prevent abuse. Washington: National Academies Press; 1985. https://www.ncbi.nlm.nih.gov.
3. Frank JW, Moore RS, Ames GM. Historical and cultural roots of drinking problems among American Indians. Am J Public Health. 2000;90(3):344–51. https://www.ncbi.nlm.nih.gov.
4. Campbell AW. Temperance movement. VCU Libraries Social Welfare History Project; 2022. https://socialwelfare.library.vcu.edu.
5. Burns K, Novick K. Roots of prohibition. WETA/PBS; 2011. https://www.pbs.org/kenburns/prohibition.
6. Editorial Staff, The MOB Museum. Women led the temperance movement. The MOB Museum: National Museum of Organized Crime & Law Enforcement; Undated. https://prohibition.themobmuseum.org.
7. NIAAA. Understanding alcohol use disorder. NIH/National Institute of Alcohol Abuse and Alcoholism; 2021. https://www.niaaa.nih.gov.
8. NIAAA. Alcohol use disorder (AUD) in the United States. NIH/National Institute of Alcohol Abuse and Alcoholism; 2023. https://www.niaaa.nih.gov.
9. Bourne M, Generes WM. Alcohol abuse in the Native American populations. American Addiction Centers; 2023. https://americanaddictioncenters.org.
10. WHO. Alcohol. World Health Organization; 2022. https://www.who.int.
11. Mayo Clinic. Alcohol use disorder. Mayo Clinic; 2022. https://wwwmayoclinic.org.
12. Rahman A. Paul M. Delirium tremens. NCBI Bookshelf: National Library of Medicine, National Institutes of Health; 2022. https://www.ncbi.nlm.nih.gov.

Opioid Use Disorder

13. Azadfard M, Huecker MR, Leaming JM. Opioid addiction. NCBI Bookshelf: National Library of Medicine, National Institutes of Health; 2023. https://www.ncbi.nlm.nih.gov.
14. NIH/NIDA. Drug overdose death rates. National Institutes of Health/National Institute on Drug Abuse; 2023. https://nida.nih.gov.
15. CDC. Understanding the opioid overdose epidemic. Centers for Disease Control and Prevention; 2022. https://www.cdc.gov.
16. Trickey E. Inside the Story of America's 19th century opiate addiction. Smithsonian Magazine. 2018. https://www.smithsonianmag.com.
17. Little B. How Civil War medicine led to America's first opioid crisis. History.com. 2021. https://www.history.com.
18. Jones JS. Opiate addiction in the Civil War's aftermath. Virginia Museum of History & Culture Magazine. 2020. https://virginiahistory.org.
19. Tackett B. History of drug use in wartime. American Addiction Centers; 2023. https://recovery.org.
20. Myers T. Panacea, poison and psychopharmacology: the lure of laudanum. J Victorian Cult Online. 2020. https://jvc.oup.com.
21. The Recovery Village. Laudanum addiction. The Recovery Village; 2022. https://www.therecoveryvillage.com.
22. Cock-Starkey C. The lure of laudanum, the Victorians' favorite drug. Mental Floss. 2023. https://www.mentalflos.com.
23. Johns Hopkins Medicine. Opioid use disorder. Johns Hopkins University; 2023. https://hopkinsmedicin.org/health.
24. Lynn RR, Galinkin JL. Naloxone dosage for opioid reversal: current evidence and clinical implications. Ther Adv Drug Saf. 2018;9(1):63–88. https://wwwncbi.nlm.nih.gov.
25. NIH/NIDA. Effective treatments for opioid addiction. National Institutes of Health/National Institute on Drug Abuse; 2016. https://nida.nih.gov.
26. SAMHSA. Medications for substance abuse disorders. Substance Abuse and Mental Health Services Administration; 2023. https://www.samhsa.gov.

Chapter 7
Parasitic Diseases

Abstract Parasitic diseases are acquired through multiple modes including contact with fecally contaminated soil, insect vectors, ingestion of contaminated food, and sexual intercourse. Historically referred to as "the disease of laziness," hookworm was the scourge of the South well into the twentieth century, now nearly eradicated by the installation of sanitary sewage disposal systems. Other parasites continue to infect Americans on a frequent basis. Often referred to as "neglected parasitic diseases," the CDC has targeted five parasitic infections prevalent in the United States as priorities for public health action, based on the pervasiveness of the infection, severity of the resultant illness, and the ability to treat and prevent the infections. These are Chagas disease, neurocysticercosis, toxocariasis, toxoplasmosis and trichomoniasis.

The parasitic diseases discussed in this chapter are: Hookworm; Chagas Disease; Neurocysticercosis; Toxocariasis; Toxoplasmosis; and Trichomoniasis.

Hookworm (*"The Disease of Laziness"*)

Often referred to as "the disease of laziness," infection with the parasitic hookworm (ancylostomiasis) was once the bane of the southeastern United States. Now largely eliminated within America's borders, the parasite still infects an estimated 576–740 million people worldwide [1].

The two species of hookworm responsible for most human infections are *Ancylostoma duodenale* and *Necator americanus* (Fig. 7.1). Together with roundworm (*Ascaris lumbricoides*) and whipworm (*Trichuris trichiura*), the three soil-transmitted helminths (parasitic worms) account for an estimated two billion worldwide infections in more than 100 countries—with the resultant malnutrition, anemia, and impaired physical and mental development causing the loss of productivity and self-sufficiency among the affected populations [2–4].

© The Author(s), under exclusive license to Springer Nature
Switzerland AG 2024
J. A. Shaw, *Historical Diseases from a Modern Perspective*,
https://doi.org/10.1007/978-3-031-52346-5_7

Fig. 7.1 Parasitic
Filariform Hookworm.
(Picture Source: https://
www.cdc.gov. CDC)

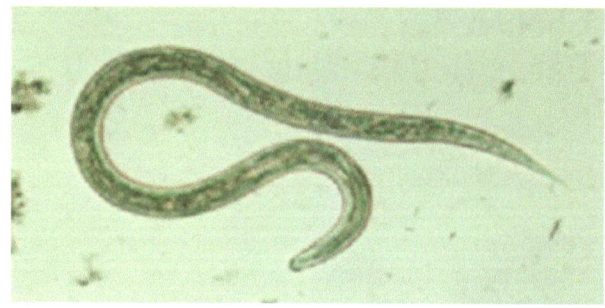

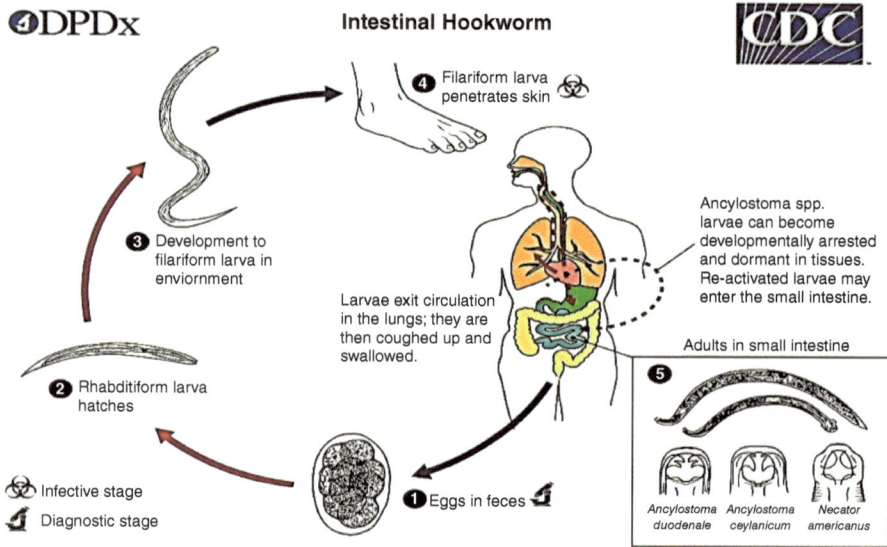

Fig. 7.2 Life Cycle of the Intestinal Hookworm. (Picture Source: https://www.cdc.gov. CDC)

Both species of human hookworm thrive in moist, hot areas where there is unsanitary disposal of human waste ("night soil"). *Necator americanus* is the predominant species in the Americas and Australia and remains endemic on islands in the Caribbean and in Central and South America [5].

Eggs from mature hookworms residing in the human small intestine are released to the environment along with feces from the infected individual. If the fecal matter is indiscriminately deposited on soil in the vicinity of human habitation (generally in the absence of an outhouse or functioning sewage disposal system) or used for garden or plant fertilizer, the eggs may mature and hatch, releasing immature worms known as rhabditiform larvae. Under appropriate environmental conditions (warm and moist soil), the immature larvae molt in 5–10 days into mature male and female filariform larvae which can penetrate the skin of humans, most commonly when people walk barefoot over infested soil (Fig. 7.2) [1, 5].

On penetration of the skin (typically bare feet), the larvae are carried through the blood vessels to the heart and then to the lungs. Upon penetrating the pulmonary alveoli, the larvae climb the bronchial tree (often creating a cough) to the pharynx where they are swallowed. When the larvae reach the jejunum of the small intestine they attach to the wall of the intestine where they mature into adult worms, mate, and produce eggs. A mature *Ancylostoma duodenale* female can produce approximately 30,000 eggs/day, the *Necator americanus* around 10,000/day [5]. Depending on the species and sex, the adult worms range in size from 5 to 15 mm long and may reside in the intestine for 1 to 2 or more years [1, 5, 6].

Although uncommon, direct ingestion of the *Ancylostoma duodenale* larvae can also cause infection. Hookworm species that infect dogs and cats cannot complete their life cycles in humans and if their larvae penetrate the skin (most commonly in the foot from fecal contaminated soil) they typically migrate within the skin creating a visible serpiginous tract, known as *cutaneous larva migrans*. Rarely, the larvae reach the gut, causing an eosinophilic enterocolitis, but do not produce eggs [1, 5].

****

Persons afflicted with hookworm infections may remain relatively asymptomatic, masking or delaying diagnosis in many cases. Penetration of the skin by the hookworm larvae may cause a foot itch ("ground itch") or a localized rash. If sufficient in number, migration of the infecting larvae through the lungs may cause coughing, wheezing, hemoptysis, and eosinophil (a type of inflammatory white cell) accumulations in the lungs and/or an increased count (number) in the peripheral blood, referred to as *Löffler Syndrome* [5, 7]. In large numbers, gut parasites may cause colicky abdominal pain, diarrhea, anorexia, and flatulence [1, 5].

Although rarely life threatening, the systemic effects of the parasitic infection are of most concern. Chronic blood loss leads to an iron deficiency anemia, weakness, fatigue, malnutrition, weight loss, and lassitude. In children the effects may be more pronounced, with heart failure, anasarca (severe peripheral edema), and impaired growth and cognitive development [1, 3–5].

Preventive measures are self-evident, but have proven difficult to implement in impoverished third world countries, with populations inured to the disease. Eliminating unhygienic defecation on soil in inhabited areas is of critical importance, with outhouses or modern sewer systems providing a surefire solution to the problem. Of equal importance, the wearing of shoes prevents penetration of the larvae into the feet, being the most common portal of bodily entry [1, 5].

Diagnosis of hookworm infections is based on the patient's clinical presentation, but most importantly on the microscopic examination of stool samples for hookworm eggs. Corroborating evidence is based on an increased eosinophil count in the peripheral blood [1, 5].

Currently, treatment of hookworm infections is relatively straightforward. Several anthelminthic drugs including albendazole, mebendazole, and pyrantel pamoate are available, effective, FDA approved and have minimal side effects [1, 5, 8]. Supportive care and iron supplement may be needed if significant anemia is present.

Under the auspices of the WHO and/or other public health organizations, mass drug administration has sometimes been used as an empirical treatment regimen for groups at risk in endemic areas, including preschool and school-age children and pregnant women [1]. The fundamental problem with such initiatives is that anthelminthic drugs only rid the patients of current infections, not future infections. As such, research and clinical testing is currently underway for hookworm vaccines using a variety of platforms [9, 10].

****

With little doubt, the infection most commonly associated with the American South is hookworm. Probably brought to the Americas via the African slave trade, the disease smoldered unrecognized for generations in the Southeast until brought to light in 1902 by Dr. Charles W. Stiles (1867–1941). Afflicting 40% (or more) of the population in some areas, it is now generally accepted that the perception of laziness, shiftlessness, and lassitude associated with people in the deep south during the nineteenth and early twentieth centuries had some basis in physiology—namely severe anemia and malnutrition caused by hookworm infections [11, 12].

As elsewhere, poverty and hookworms were inexorably linked in the Deep South. City dwellers, plantation owners, and persons of means wore shoes, used chamber pots and outhouses or, in later years, had indoor plumbing. Poor folks and slaves frequently went barefoot, defecated in rudimentary or overflowing latrines or in the woods. Fecal slop was used for fertilizer on land worked by slaves or sharecroppers, spreading infection among those of lower economic status and perpetuating the infection-related stigmata of laziness and inferiority.[1]

It is hard to imagine a whole segment of the U.S. population afflicted with a parasite that sapped them of energy, while remaining totally ignorant (or accepting) of their plight. Astonishingly, that was the case until 1902 when Dr. Stiles (Fig. 7.3) recognized similar lethargic symptoms in the impoverished people of the South that he had observed abroad during his research on intestinal parasites [11].

After identifying a new species of hookworm, *Uncinaria americana* (later named *Necator americanus*), afflicting the Southerners, Stiles sought financial aid from John D. Rockefeller, who was searching for a philanthropic project. Together they established the Rockefeller Sanitary Commission for the Eradication of Hookworm Disease (1909–1914) which worked feverishly with state and local governments to help eradicate the scourge of hookworm [11–13].

Spanning 11 southern states, Stile's initiative extended education to healthcare providers, teachers, and the populous at large, and in the process strove to minimize the offensive social stigmata associated with the disease. Preventive measures such as the construction of sanitary latrines and the routine wearing of shoes were emphasized and over 400,000 people were treated for the affliction [11].

By today's standards the medical treatment of hookworm infections in the early 1900s was somewhat archaic. One of the earliest pharmaceuticals used was Thymol [14, 15]. A component of thyme oil, the medication was given in age-titrated doses with varying proportions of lactose and sodium bicarbonate or, in accordance with

---

[1]An interesting history of the South's hookworm infestation, with personal anecdotes, is given in Rachel Nuwer's Nova/PBS account: *How a Worm Gave the South a Bad Name* (http://www.pbs.org).

Fig. 7.3 Charles W. Stiles, PhD (1867–1941). (Picture Source: https://www.nal. usda.gov. USDA National Agriculture Library)

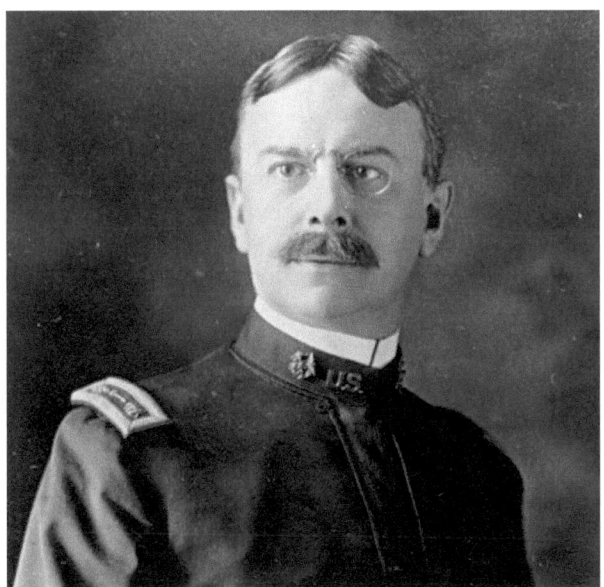

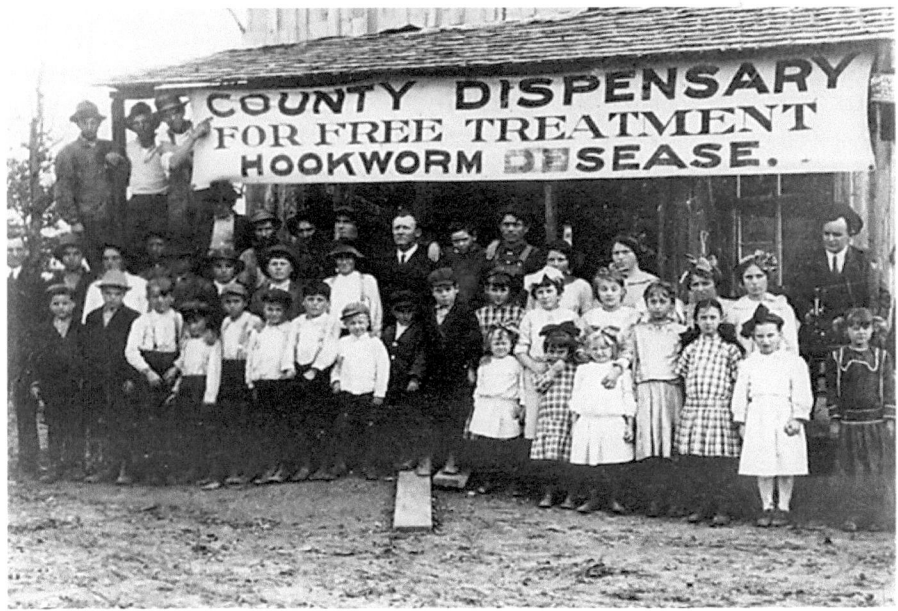

Fig. 7.4 Dispensary for free hookworm treatment. Faulkner County, Arkansas. Circa 1912. (Picture Source: https://www.npr.org. Getty Images)

Dr. Stiles' recommendation, in conjunction with a pre-dosing purgative of Epsom salts [15]. Treatment was followed a few days later by microscopic stool examination to determine if a cure had been realized. Repeated dosing was often needed (Fig. 7.4).

Found to be considerably more efficacious, carbon tetrachloride was introduced in the early 1920s by Dr. Maurice C. Hall (1881–1938) for the treatment of hookworm. Along with tetrachloroethylene, which Dr. Hall also introduced, both drugs played a vital role in the virtual eradication of hookworm in the USA [16, 17]. Administered orally in small amounts, both medications were readily tolerated and remarkably effective anthelmintics, typically requiring only a single-dose regimen. However, with concerns about liver toxicity and potential carcinogenicity, both compounds have been replaced by the modern drugs mentioned previously and are principally used in dry cleaning, textile processing, and degreasing applications at this time.

Facing patient and physician apathy and, at times, open hostility, together with a lack of money and time, the Rockefeller Sanitary Commission never achieved its lofty goal of eliminating hookworm from the South [18]. However, with ever-improving sewage disposal systems, continued public awareness campaigns and more efficacious medications, the incidence of hookworm infections dropped over ensuing decades to the point that the International Health Board (IHB) declared the disease eradicated in the South in 1927 [18].

Be that as it may, subsequent studies have identified pockets of persistent hookworm in the southern states [18]. Most recently, a 2017 study published in the *American Journal of Tropical Medicine and Hygiene* uncovered a community of people infected with hookworm in rural Alabama [19]. An impoverished area with inadequate and overflowing septic systems, often with raw sewage backing into their houses, residents were particularly susceptible to hookworm infections, according to the study's authors. Nineteen of the 55 persons tested were positive for the worm.

This and other studies point out the need for constant vigilance, continuing education, and improved sanitary infrastructure implementation and maintenance—both here and abroad—to eliminate this eminently preventable disease as a continuing source of human misery.

Neglected Parasitic Diseases

A general perception within the USA is that parasitic infections are exclusively found in poor and underdeveloped countries. Nothing could be further from the truth. As ancient as mankind itself, parasitic infections are common in America, affecting millions in some cases. They can cause serious illness, including seizures, blindness, cardiac failure, and death. Persons living in poor or disadvantaged neighborhoods are at greatest risk, many not knowing they are infected [20].

Fortunately, most parasitic infections can be successfully treated with antiparasitic drugs or antibiotics if recognized early in the course of active infection. Unfortunately, many persons do not avail themselves of treatment, either not realizing they are infected or not having ready access to medical care. Often primary care providers are unfamiliar with parasitic infections and may not make timely diagnoses or treat them appropriately [20, 21].

The CDC has targeted five parasitic infections prevalent in the USA as priorities for public health action, based on the pervasiveness of the infection, severity of the resultant illness, and the ability to treat and prevent the infections. These are Chagas disease, neurocysticercosis, toxocariasis, toxoplasmosis, and trichomoniasis [20, 21].

Often grouped as "neglected parasitic infections," none of the five have received the massive public health initiatives for eradication which were focused on hookworm and malaria in the past, as outlined in previous sections. Discussed only in brief below, the reader is encouraged to explore the many excellent online references written for the general public on each of these common infections.

****

- **Chagas disease** is a parasitic infection caused by the protozoan *Trypanosoma cruzi*. First identified by Brazilian physician Carlos Chagas (1879–1934) in 1909, the disease is endemic in Latin America and is most commonly found in the USA among persons who are recent immigrants.

  The WHO estimates that 6–7 million people worldwide are infected with the Chagas parasite [22]. In 2022 the CDC estimated that there were 300,000 persons carrying the parasite within the States, most of whom are unaware of their infection [23].

  The *T. cruzi* parasite is principally transmitted to humans through the feces of the blood-sucking insect known as the triatomine bug (Fig. 7.5). Often referred to as the "kissing bug," the infected triatomine commonly defecates near the site of a bite wound, most often inflicted during the night when a person is sleeping. The fecally deposited *T. cruzi* parasites gain entrance to their human hosts through the bite wound or through mucosal membranes when the human host scratches a bite and then inadvertently transfers the insect's feces to his or her eyes or mouth. Alternate pathways of transmission include blood transfusions, organ transplants, and mother-to-child (congenital) transmission [23].

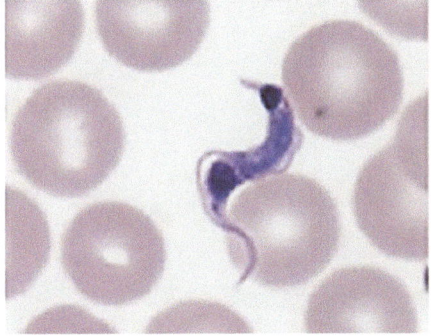 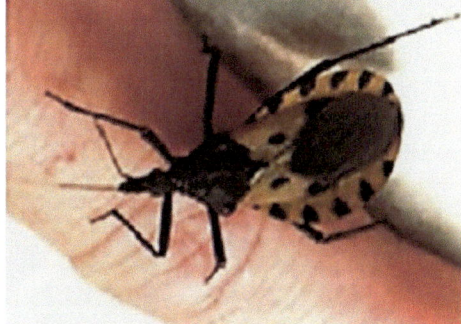

Fig. 7.5 *T. cruzi* parasite (left) transmitted by the triatomine bug (right). (Picture Source: https://www.cdc.gov/parasites/chagas. CDC: DPDx)

Without treatment, approximately 20–30% of infected persons develop cardiac, intestinal, or neurological complications including cardiomegaly (enlarged heart), heart failure, arrhythmias, cardiac arrest (death), megaesophagus, megacolon, and peripheral neuropathy [22, 23].

Treatment in the early stages of the disease with the antiparasitic drugs, Benznidazole and Nifurtimox, is very effective with a cure rate approaching 100% [24]. Treatment of chronic infections is generally non-curative but may curb symptomatic disease progression and prevent transmission [22]. There are no vaccines available for Chagas disease at this time.

- **Neurocysticercosis** is a parasitic infection caused by ingestion of the eggs from the adult pork tapeworm, *Taenia solium*. Larval cysts (oncospheres) mature from the ingested eggs and cross the intestinal mucosa where they migrate through the bloodstream to the brain, muscles, and eyes, among other structures. Once in the brain, the cysts may remain viable for years, causing the clinical syndrome referred to as neurocysticercosis (Fig. 7.6) [20, 25, 26].

  Neurocysticercosis is the principal cause of infective seizures in the developing world and with the ever-increasing migration of persons from Latin America to the USA, it has become increasingly prevalent in America. Based on 2020 data, the CDC estimates that there are 1000 new hospitalizations for neurocysticercosis in the USA each year [20].

  The diagnosis of neurocysticercosis is based on the patient's clinical presentation, history of possible tapeworm egg exposure, imaging studies (CT/MRI), and serology testing. Treatment varies depending on the severity and duration of symptoms, with anticonvulsant therapy the mainstay of management for the

Fig. 7.6 Radiographic image of *T. solium* larval cysts in the brain. (Picture Source: https://www.cdc.gov/parasites/cysticerosis. CDC)

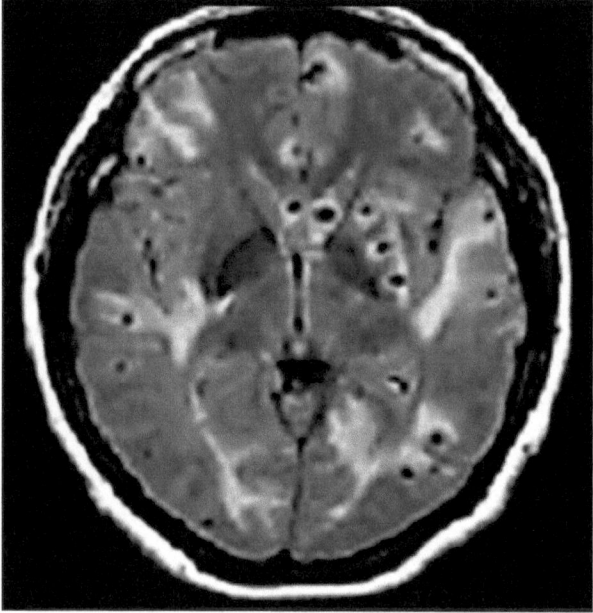

associated seizures. Anthelmintic therapy (albendazole and praziquantel) is generally indicated for symptomatic patients with multiple, live (noncalcified) cysticerci [25, 27].

Prevention of neurocysticercosis is based on initiatives to raise global awareness, encouraging thorough hand-washing hygiene and treatment of existing intestinal tapeworms.

- **Toxocariasis** is caused by infection with the larvae of the dog and cat roundworm, *Toxocara canis* and *Toxocara cati*, respectively. These roundworms are the most ubiquitous intestinal nematode parasites of dogs and cats. Transmission of the parasite to humans generally occurs when an infected dog or cat sheds *Toxocara* eggs in their feces into environmental soil. Eggs are subsequently transferred to the human host by touching a soil/fecal/egg contaminated hand to the mouth during gardening, disposing of pet waste or, most commonly, during outdoor child-play with pet dogs or cats [20, 28, 29].

  Once ingested, roundworm larvae hatch from the eggs and migrate to various parts of the body through the bloodstream. Two principal forms of toxocariasis are the most common. Ocular toxocariasis (ocular larva migrans) occurs when the larvae migrate to the eye, potentially causing visual impairment and blindness, typically involving only one eye. Visceral toxocariasis (visceral larva migrans) occurs when the larvae migrate to the liver, lungs or other organs, with symptoms commensurate with the organ involved [29–31].

  Antibody testing suggests that millions of Americans have been exposed to *Toxocara*, although most remain asymptomatic. The CDC estimates that 70 people, mostly children, are blinded by toxocariasis every year in the United States [20].

  As with other parasite infections, diagnosis is based on the presenting symptoms and signs, exposure history, and serological testing. When indicated, treatment may include the antiparasitic medicines albendazole and mebendazole, steroids to reduce inflammation and occasionally surgery in ocular cases [30, 31].

  Prevention of toxocariasis is based on controlling *Toxocara* infections in dogs and cats by deworming, reducing risk of larvae contact by proper handling and disposal of dog and cat feces, and hand washing before food preparation and after playing with pets [20].

- **Toxoplasmosis** is an endemic parasitic infection in the USA caused by the protozoan parasite, *Toxoplasma gondii*. The CDC estimates suggest that 11% of the U.S. population over 6 years of age have been infected with *Toxoplasma* [32].

  Most infected persons have little or no symptoms and do not require treatment. Others may experience mild symptoms including fever, malaise, and swollen lymph nodes. A small percentage suffer retinal eye disease, while infection during pregnancy may result in a miscarriage or developmental delays, blindness or epilepsy in the newborn [20, 33].

  Infected persons generally remain infected for life, which places persons with immune compromise (HIV, cancer, organ transplant, etc.) at risk for reactivation of quiescent parasites with a propensity to affect the lungs, brain, and central nervous system. Symptoms may include respiratory distress, headache, seizures, facial paralysis, encephalitis, coma, and death [20, 34].

Although most mammals can harbor the *T. gondii* parasite, only cats can shed environmentally resistant cysts (oocysts) in their feces. As such, one of the common modes of human transmission is ingesting food, soil or water contaminated with cat feces, typically via unwashed fruits and vegetables, or hand-to-mouth contact following gardening or cleaning a cat's litter box (Fig. 7.7) [20].

Other modes of transmission are eating raw or undercooked meat containing parasitic tissue cysts or congenital mother-to-fetus transfer (transplacental transmission) during pregnancy. Transfer during an organ transplant or blood transfusion from an infected person to an uninfected person is also possible [20, 35].

As with other parasitic infections, diagnosis is generally based on the clinical presentation, history of possible cyst exposure, and serology testing. Histological examination of infecting cysts, polymerase chain reaction (PCR) of bodily fluids, and parasite culture are also possible [33].

While antibiotics (sulfadiazine and pyrimethamine) and steroids are helpful in treating ophthalmologic disease, prevention through education, proper food

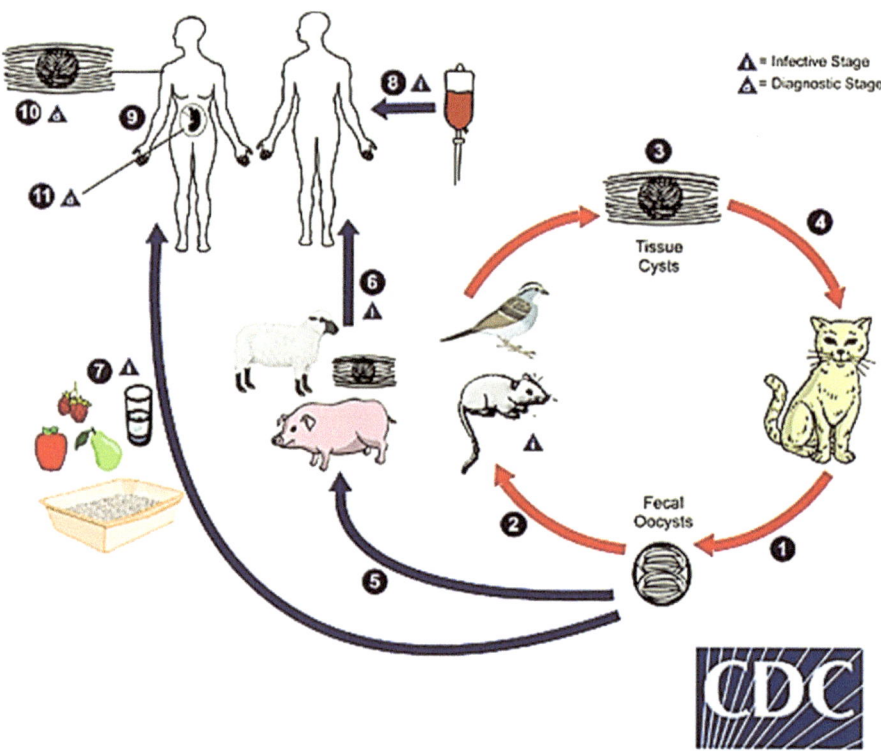

Fig. 7.7 Transmission modes the *T. gondii* parasite. (Picture Source: https://www.cdc.gov/parasites/toxoplasmosi. CDC)

preparation, hand washing, and appropriate handling and disposal of cat litter remain the mainstay of *Toxoplasma gondii* parasite control [20, 33].

- **Trichomoniasis** (*"trich"*) is one of the most prevalent sexually transmitted diseases (STDs) in the USA. Caused by the protozoan parasite, *Trichomonas vaginalis* (Fig. 7.8), approximately 3.7 million persons are infected in America according to CDC estimates [20].

  Women infected with *T. vaginalis* may experience vaginal discharge, painful intercourse, vaginal itching, and pelvic pain. Similarly, men may exhibit penile discharge, urinary frequency, dysuria, and testicular pain. That said, a majority of infected persons remain asymptomatic, making recognition of infection problematic and enhancing the likelihood of continued transmission, totally unawares. Pregnant women with trich are prone to deliver their children prematurely and with low birth weights [36, 37].

  The diagnosis of *Trichomonas* infections is based on history, physical examination (e.g., "strawberry cervix"), wet prep microscopy to identify the flagellated organisms, and culture of vaginal or penile exudate. Nucleic acid amplification tests are also available with high sensitivity and specificity [36, 37].

  Some untreated cases of trichomoniasis may remain subclinical or resolve with the host's immune response. However, antibiotic treatment (metronidazole) is highly recommended with a cure rate of 90–95% [36]. Of note, reinfection is likely if the sexual partner is not treated simultaneously. Moreover, untreated persons have been shown to have a higher risk of acquiring and transmitting other STDs, including HIV, adding imperativeness to curative antibiotic treatment [20, 36].

Fig. 7.8 *Trichomonas vaginalis* parasites. (Picture Source: https://www.cdc.gov/std/trichomonas. CDC)

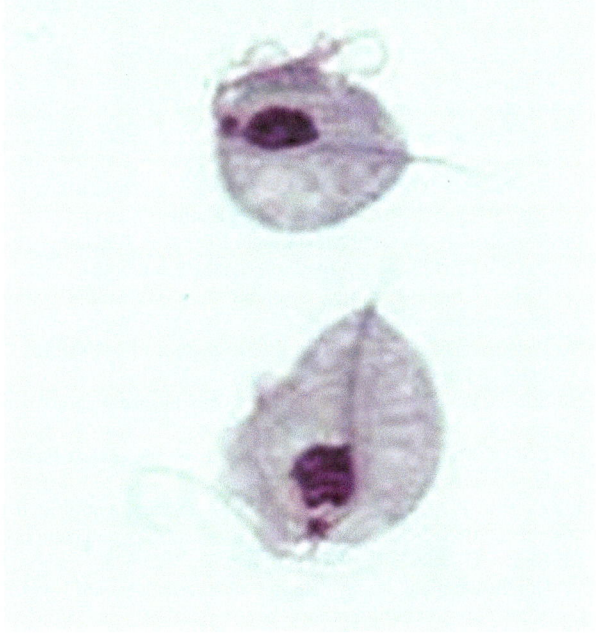

Prevention and control of *Trichomonas* infection transmission is focused on patient education, treatment of concurrent sexual partners, and use of barrier contraception. Follow-up screening after treatment is imperative to ensure a complete cure.

References

Hookworm

1. CDC. Parasites—hookworm. Centers for Disease Control and Prevention; 2020. https://www.cdc.gov.
2. WHO. Eliminating soil-transmitted helminthiases as a public health problem in children. In: Progress report 2001-2010 and strategic plan 2011-2020. World Health Organization; 2012. https://www.who.int.
3. Becker SL, Liwanag HJ, Snyder JS, et al. Toward the 2020 goal of soil-transmitted helminthiasis control and elimination. PLoS Negl Trop Dis. 2018;12(8):e0006606. https://www.ncbi.nlm.nih.gov.
4. Kuong K, Fiorentino M, Perignon M, et al. Cognitive performance and iron status are negatively associated with hookworm infection in Cambodian schoolchildren. Am J Trop Med Hyg. 2016;95(4):856–63. https://www.ncbi.nlm.nih.gov.
5. Marie C, Petri WA. Hookworm infection. Merck Manual: professional version. 2022. https://www.merckmanuals.com.
6. Kliegman RM. Hookworms (*Necator americanus* and *Ancylostoma* spp.). In: Nelson textbook of pediatrics. Amsterdam: Elsevier; 2020. https://www.sciencedirect.com.
7. Sharma GD. Loffler syndrome. Medscape. 2022. https://emedicine.medscape.com.
8. Malik K, Dua A. Albendazole. StatPearls-NCBI Bookshelf: National Library of Medicine, National Institutes of Health; 2022. https://www.ncbi.nlm.nih.gov.
9. Hotez PJ, Diemert D, Bacon KM, et al. The human hookworm vaccine. Vaccine. 2013;31(2):227–32. https://www.ncbi.nlm.nih.gov.
10. Chapman PR, Webster R, Giacomin P. Vaccination of human participants with attenuated *Necator americanus* hookworm larvae and human challenge in Australia: a dose-finding study and randomized, placebo-controlled, phase 1 trial. The Lancet. 2021;21(12):1725–36. https://www.thelancet.com.
11. Sanders JW, Goraleski KA. The hookworm blues: we still got em. Am J Trop Med Hyg. 2017;97(5):1277–9. https://www.ncbi.nlm.nih.gov.
12. Schneider B, Jariwala AR, Periago MV, et al. A history of vaccine development. Hum Vaccin. 2011;7(11):1234–44. https://www.ncbi.nlm.nih.gov.
13. USDA. Charles w. Stiles. Special collections, USDA National Agriculture Library; Undated. https://www.nal.usda.gov.
14. Washburn BE. Use of thymol in treatment of hookworm disease. JAMA. 1917;LXVIII(16):1162–3. https://jamanetwork.com.
15. Stiles CW. The treatment of hookworm disease. Public Health Rep. 1909;24:34. https://www.jstor.org.
16. USDA. Maurice C. Hall. Special collections, USDA National Agriculture Library; Undated. https://www.nal.usda.gov.
17. Lamson PD, Minot AS, Robins BH. The prevention and treatment of carbon tetrachloride intoxication. JAMA. 1928;90(5):345–9. https://jamanetwork.com.
18. Elman C, McGuire RA, Wittman B. Extending public health: the Rockefeller Sanitary Commission and hookworm in the American South. Am J Public Health. 2014;104(1):47–58. https://www.ncbi.nlm.nih.gov.

19. McKenna ML, McAtee S, Bryan PE, et al. Human intestinal parasite burden and poor sanitation in rural Alabama. Am J Trop Med Hyg. 2017;97(5):1623–8. https://www.ajtmh.org.

Neglected Parasitic Infections

20. CDC. Neglected parasitic infections in the United States. Centers for Disease Control and Prevention; 2020. https://www.cdc.gov.
21. Hotez PJ. Neglected parasitic infections and poverty in the United States. PLoS Negl Trop Dis. 2014;8(9):e3012. https://www.ncbi.nlm.nih.gov.
22. WHO. Chagas disease (also known as American trypanosomiasis). World Health Organization; 2023. https://who.int.
23. CDC. Parasites—American trypanosomiasis (also known as Chagas disease). Centers for Disease Control and Prevention; 2022. https://www.cdc.gov.
24. PAHO/WHO. Chagas disease: Pan American Health Organization. 2022. https://www.paho.org.
25. DeGiorgio CM, Medina MT, Duron R, et al. Neurocysticercosis. Epilepsy Curr. 2004;4(3):107–11. https://www.ncbi.nl,.nih.gov.
26. Garcia HH, Del Nash TE, Brutto OH. Clinical symptoms, diagnosis, and treatment of neurocysticercosis. Lancet Neurol. 2014;13(2):1202–15. https://www.ncbi.nlm.nih.gov.
27. CDC. Parasites—cysticercosis: resources for health professionals. Centers for Disease Control and Prevention; 2020. https://www.cdc.gov.
28. Chen J, Liu Q, Liu G-H, et al. A silent threat with a progressive public health impact. Infect Dis Poverty. 2018;7(9):59. https://idpjournal.biomedcentral.com.
29. Woodhall DM, Eberhard ML, Parise ME. Neglected parasitic infections in the United States: toxocariasis. Am J Trop Med Hyg. 2014;90(5):810–3. https://www.ncbi.nlm.nih.gov.
30. CDC. Parasites—toxocariasis (also known as roundworm infection): resources for health professionals. Centers for Disease Control and Prevention; 2020. https://www.cdc.gov.
31. Ahn SJ, Ryoo N-K, Woo SJ. Ocular toxocariasis: clinical features, diagnosis, treatment, and prevention. Asia Pac Allergy. 2014;4(3):134–41. https://www.ncbi.nlm.nih.gov.
32. CDC. Parasites—toxoplasmosis (toxoplasma infection): epidemiology & risk factors. Centers for Disease Control and Prevention; 2018. https://www.cdc.gov.
33. Furtado JM, Smith JR, Belfort R Jr, et al. Toxoplasmosis: a global threat. J Global Infect Dis. 2011;3(3):281–4. https://www.ncbi.nlm.nih.gov.
34. Mayo Clinic. Toxoplasmosis. Mayo Clinic; 2023. https://www.mayoclinic.org.
35. CDC. Parasites—toxoplasmosis (toxoplasma infection): biology. Centers for Disease Control and Prevention; 2020. https://www.cdc.gov.
36. Schumann JA, Plasner S. Trichomoniasis. In: StatPearls. New York: National Institutes of Health; 2022. https://www.ncbi.nlm.nih.gov.
37. CDC. Trichomoniasis—CDC basic fact sheet. Centers for Disease Control and Prevention; 2022. https://www.cdc.gov.

Chapter 8
Nutritional Diseases

Abstract The two nutritional diseases of major historical impact discussed in this chapter are rickets and scurvy, caused by a deficiency of vitamins D and C, respectively. The ravages of scurvy decimated sailors, polar explorers, and armies on the move in the years before citrus fruits were identified as preventative and curative. Rickets was a pervasive scourge on society, particularly in northern climes, until cod liver oil was fortuitously identified as preventative, and vitamin D fortification was subsequently introduced into milk and other food staples in the 1930s. The pathophysiology of rickets and scurvy is discussed in some detail.

Vitamin D Deficiency (*Rickets*)

Possibly deriving its name from the German word "wricken" (meaning "twisted") [1], rickets is a childhood disease of bone caused by a lack of vitamin D, calcium, or phosphorus, which results in softened and inadequately mineralized bones. Bone deformities, including bowed legs, breastbone projection, thickened wrists and ankles, knobby ribs, spine curvatures, misshapen skulls, and generalized growth retardation are common to varying degrees (Fig. 8.1). Muscle weakness, bone pain, tetany, poor dentition, and delayed motor skills may also be associated with the disease [2, 3].

Most commonly, rickets results from a dietary deficiency in vitamin D (nutritional rickets), but may also be caused by insufficient exposure to sunlight or a variety of genetic disorders, liver or kidney diseases, medications, and malabsorption syndromes [2, 3].

Bone is composed of a protein matrix (osteoid) upon which a ceramic-like compound of calcium and phosphorus (hydroxyapatite) is deposited to form a composite structure. The inorganic minerals provide the bone's strength and rigidity, the organic osteoid the bone's formative template [4].

Fig. 8.1 Child exhibiting
bowed legs, characteristic
of rickets. Wadesboro, NC,
1938. (Picture Source:
https://www.gettyimages.
CORBIS Historical:
Library of Congress)

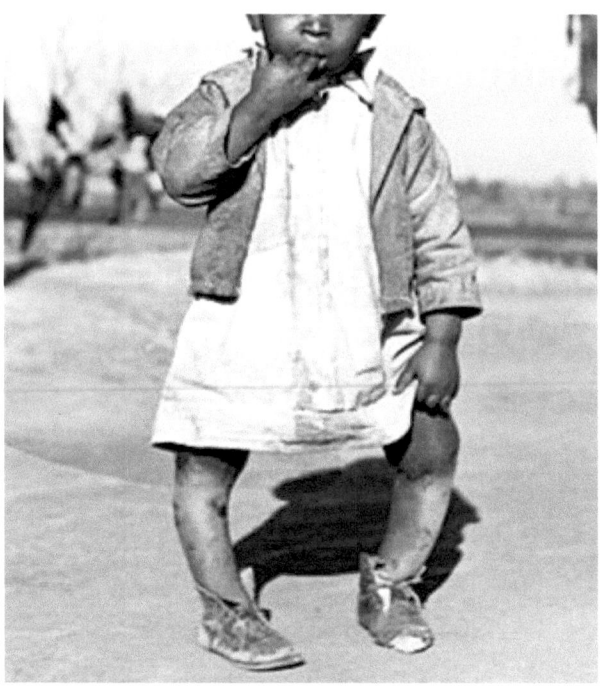

In addition to its role in the structure of bone, calcium plays an essential role in neuromuscular physiology, cardiac contractility, and blood clotting. A low calcium blood level can lead to tetany or seizures, as well. If blood calcium levels fall too low due to inadequate dietary intake or poor gut absorption, the parathyroid gland releases a hormone (parathormone) which activates bone resorbing cells (osteoclasts). These cells liberate calcium from the bones into the serum to restore appropriate blood calcium levels [4]. If the bone matrix loses sufficient structural calcium and phosphorus, the bones become soft, deformable, and prone to fracture—a state referred to as rickets in children. The same cascade of metabolic events in adults, called osteomalacia, results in weakened bones (lacking mineral content) with a propensity to fracture, but rarely causes deformity unless pre-existing.

Although the lack of dietary calcium and phosphorus may be a contributing cause of rickets, the principal cause in most cases is the lack of vitamin D [2, 3]. Vitamin D is a hormone that facilitates the absorption of calcium and phosphorus in the gut, which are otherwise poorly absorbed. Without adequate amounts of vitamin D, blood and bone levels of calcium and phosphorus are likely to remain low even if the dietary intake of the two minerals (which are found in multiple food groups) would otherwise be sufficient to maintain normal circulating blood levels and bone mineralization.

Vitamin D is available to the body through two routes. The first is an endogenous route via the action of the sun's rays on skin [5, 6]. Ultraviolet light penetrating the epidermal layer of the skin converts an endogenously formed precursor vitamin (7-dehydrocholesterol) into vitamin D-3 (cholecalciferol). The D-3 vitamin is further modified in the liver and kidney into more active forms, 25-hydroxy vitamin D and 1,25-dihydroxy vitamin D, collectively referred to as vitamin D. The second is an exogenous route via direct dietary intake of vitamin D [2, 3].

There are problems intrinsic to both pathways, which may result in insufficient levels of vitamin D and the development of rickets or osteomalacia [2, 3]. Genetic abnormalities may interfere with the metabolic pathways essential to the formation of vitamin D. Similarly, liver or kidney diseases may hamper the transformation of vitamin D-3 into its more active forms. But the most common cause of insufficient endogenously produced vitamin D is inadequate exposure to sunlight, most notably in northern climes during winter months, particularly among those who work (or play) indoors during daylight hours or are confined to their homes for extended periods due to prevailing weather conditions, physical disabilities, or psycho-social isolation. Persons of dark skin pigmentation are particularly vulnerable because the melanin in the skin blocks ultraviolet light penetration, limiting vitamin D-3 production (while also reducing damaging effects of sunlight on skin, including skin cancer)—possibly explaining the evolutionary transition from dark to light skin in humans residing in northern regions of the world [1, 7].

Adequate dietary intake of vitamin D is problematic for the simple reason that the vitamin is not present in many foods. Fruits and vegetables do not contain vitamin D. Most meats have little or no vitamin D. Fatty fish, egg yolks, and some mushrooms are the principal sources of naturally occurring vitamin D, which may not form a large portion of many people's diets [2, 3].

Without any fundamental understanding of its mechanism of action, cod liver oil was anecdotally identified as a curative therapy for rickets in the mid-1800s [8]. With advertisements (Fig. 8.2) claiming *"A well-shaped head ... A fine, full chest ... A strong back ... Straight legs ... Strong, even teeth,"* the oil became the mainstay of

Fig. 8.2 1940 Squibb advertisement for cod liver oil. (Picture Source: https://www.etsy.com. Squibb Corporation)

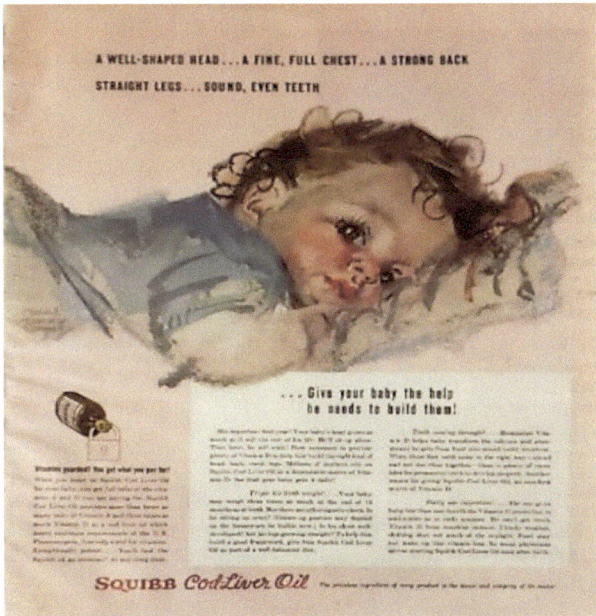

science-supported preventive nutrition following the identification of vitamin D by Sir Edward Mellanby (1884–1995) and others in the early 1900s [1, 9], and the subsequent chemical analysis of cod liver oil revealing its abundant concentration of vitamin D—then recognized as essential for the absorption of calcium and phosphorus in the gut.

· With the isolation of vitamin D precursors in some plants and fungi (yeast) and animal (pig) skin in the 1930s, fortification of foods (milk, orange juice, dairy products, cereals, infant formula, etc.) with vitamin D became possible, virtually eliminating the scourge of rickets in the USA and many other countries [10].

****

Unfortunately, there has been an uptick of rickets in the USA in recent years, the cause of which is thought to be multifactorial [1, 11, 12]. Breast milk does not contain enough vitamin D to prevent rickets in isolation and the trend in recent decades away from infant formula toward prolonged and exclusive breast feeding may be partially responsible. Indoor childhood play glued to computers and video games may limit outdoor activities and sunlight exposure, as may the liberal use of sunscreen and protective clothing to guard against skin cancer. A transition away from milk consumption (which is high in calcium and fortified with vitamin D) toward soda and/or bottled water may also be a contributing factor, as may a transition toward vegetarian diets.

As the exposure time to sunlight necessary to prevent rickets is poorly defined and highly variable with respect to latitude, season, climate, age, and skin pigmentation, coupled with real concerns referable to sun exposure and skin cancer, dietary supplementation with vitamin D is generally recommended to prevent rickets and osteomalacia at this time. Daily recommendations vary but center around 10 mcg (400 IU) for infants up to 1 year of age and 15 mcg (600 IU) for older children and adults [1, 13]. Larger doses may be recommended for the elderly and pregnant or lactating women.

Vitamin C Deficiency (*Scurvy*)

With the exception of obesity [14], nutritional diseases are relatively uncommon in the USA at this time. But, any student of history or fan of historical novels knows that scurvy was a major cause of disability and mortality among early global sailors and polar explorers.[1]

---

[1]The reader might enjoy reading: Laurence Bergreen's book *Over the Edge of the World: Magellan's Terrifying Circumnavigation of the Globe* (HarperCollins Publishers, New York, NY, 2003) and/or Fergus Fleming's book *Ninety Degrees North: The Quest for the North Pole* (Granta Books, London, England, 2001).

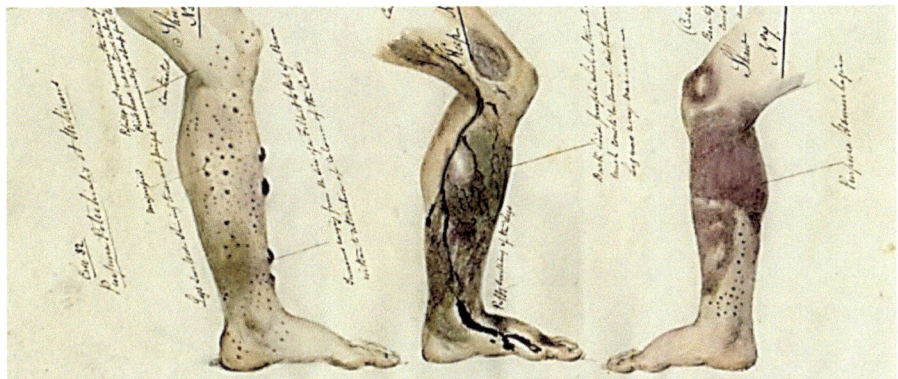

Fig. 8.3 Watercolor illustrations of scurvy signs. Circa 1841. Henry W. Mahon. (Picture Source: https://www.sciencehistory.org. The National Archives, UK)

Scurvy is caused by a lack of dietary vitamin C (ascorbic acid), plentifully found in fresh fruits and vegetables. Unlike most other mammals who require no dietary source, vitamin C is an essential (exogenously acquired) dietary vitamin in humans. Vitamin C plays a critical role in the formation of collagen and the lack of the vitamin interferes with normal tissue synthesis [15].

Vitamin C deficiency causes lethargy, weight loss, weakness, anemia, gum disease, and skin hemorrhages. Symptomatic scurvy develops after several months of dietary deficiency. Bleeding manifests itself as skin bruises or may occur around lower extremity skin follicles or into joints (Fig. 8.3). Gums often become swollen and spongy, and teeth may loosen and fall out. Hair characteristically becomes brittle and coils into a "corkscrew-like" configuration or may simply fall out. Legs often become edematous and skin scaly. Wounds fail to heal and death may ensue from resultant infections or from internal bleeding [15, 16].

Ancient seafarers suffered terribly from scurvy. More than 2 million sailors died from scurvy between the sixteenth and mid-nineteenth centuries, by some estimates [17]. On long voyages it was an accepted reality that there would be a 50% loss of men to scurvy. Notably, in 1744 Commodore George Anson returned to port after a four-year global circumnavigation with only 188 of his 1854 crew still alive, most having succumbed to the ravages of scurvy [17, 18].[2]

Appalled by the Anson disaster, Royal Navy surgeon James Lind (1716–1794) undertook a rigorous scientific study to identify a curative remedy for scurvy while aboard the naval ship *Salisbury* in 1747 (Fig. 8.4). He determined that ingestion of citrus fruits (oranges and lemons) was both curative and preventative. His results were published in 1753, but were initially met with skepticism for a variety of reasons, both practical and philosophical.

---

[2] The Anson disaster and the ravages of scurvy are graphically described in *The Wager: A Tale of Shipwreck, Mutiny and Murder* (Doubleday, New York, NY, 2023) by David Grann.

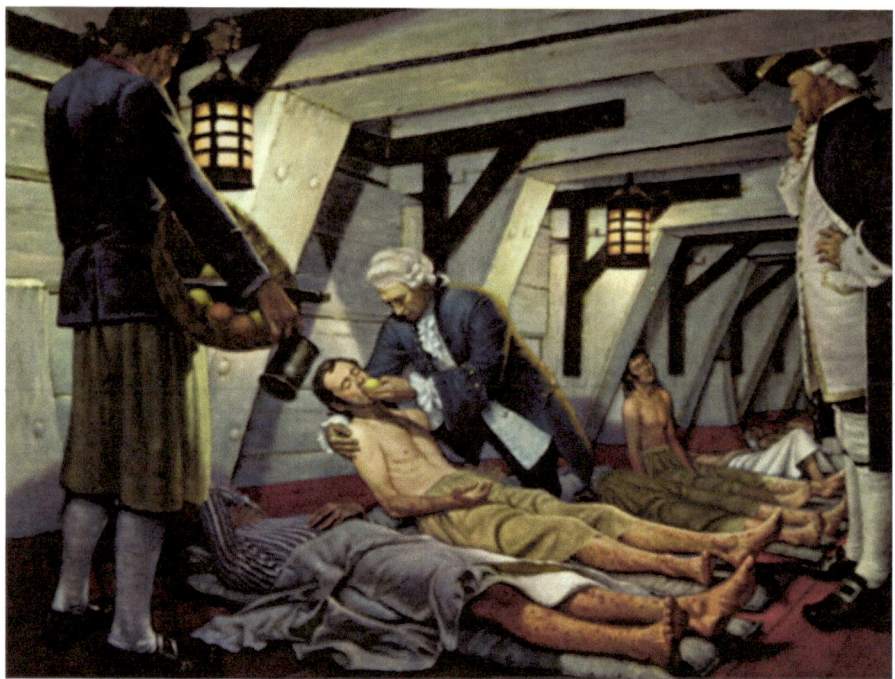

Fig. 8.4 Dr. Lind administering citrus fruit aboard the Salisbury in 1747. Artist: Robert A. Thom/ Contributor: Park-Davis & Company. (Picture Source: https://collections.nlm.nih.gov. National Library of Medicine)

Be that as it may, Lind's recommendations were ultimately adopted by the Royal Navy in 1795, mandating that three-quarters of an ounce of lemon juice (subsequently switched to lime juice based on availability) be given to every sailor on a daily basis, virtually eliminating the scourge of scurvy within the British navy. Other countries were slower on the uptake, often ridiculing the British sailors as "limeys," a term that persists to date [17–19].

In addition to besetting seafarers and polar explorers [20], scurvy has also afflicted landsmen throughout history, often among populations suffering from famine or among soldiers surviving on restricted/inadequate diets during extended military campaigns. Scurvy significantly impacted the Irish during the Great Famine of 1845–1852, caused by the precipitous decline of dietary vitamin C with the decimation of the potato crop [21]. In America, soldiers suffered most notably during the Civil War [22]. Fresh fruits and vegetables were difficult to come by, store without rotting, and transport over long distances, effectively limiting soldier's diets to repetitive rations of hard tack and salted beef and pork.

In an attempt to provide a balanced diet during the American Civil War, a product called "desiccated vegetables" was issued to troops. The product was a mixture of dried vegetables (potatoes, cabbage, turnip, carrots, parsnips, beets, tomatoes, onions, peas, beans, lentils, and celery) which were pressed into hard blocks and then dried in large ovens. Necessitating hours of boiling to soften and reconstitute and, apparently, of foul taste, soldiers often refused to eat the product, referring to it as "desecrated vegetables." Moreover, any vitamin benefits the dried concoction may have provided were likely depleted by the long cooking time necessary to make the product palatable [23].

The dietary end result during the Civil War was a nearly universal affliction of malnutrition, in general, and scurvy, in particular, among soldiers on both sides of the conflict. Prisoners-of-war camps were most severely impacted, with scurvy deaths accounting for up to 25% of prisoner mortalities. Unaccounted for were the detrimental effects of vitamin C deficiency on wound healing, which undoubtedly cost lives as well [22, 23].

****

The knowledge that scurvy is caused by a vitamin deficiency evolved over time and was not universally accepted until 1928 when Albert Szent-Györgyi (1893–1986) isolated a substance from adrenal glands that he called "hexuronic acid," later renamed to "ascorbic acid" for its anti-scorbutic (scurvy-fighting) properties. Four years later (1932), Charles Glen King (1896–1988) isolated ascorbic acid (vitamin C) in his laboratory and in 1933 Norman Haworth (1883–1950) identified its chemical structure [24].

As noted previously, vitamin C is required for the synthesis of collagen, a protein component of connective tissue which plays an essential role during wound healing. It is also now known that vitamin C is a powerful antioxidant and may play a role in limiting certain cancers, heart disease, and other afflictions where oxidant tension may be causally related [25, 26].

Today, vitamin C deficiency is rare in developed countries and overt deficiency occurs only when intake falls below 10 mg/day over many weeks [26]. Fruits and vegetables contain more than adequate amounts of vitamin C for most dietary needs, but a vitamin shortage may occur in individuals consuming a limited dietary variety, including food faddists, the elderly, and people who abuse alcohol or drugs. Infants fed only canned mild or boiled cow's milk may be at risk, as are smokers and persons with chronic diseases or malabsorption syndromes [26].

References

Vitamin D Deficiency

1. Wheeler BJ, Snoody AME, Munns C, et al. A brief history of nutritional rickets. Front Endocrinol. 2019;10. https://www.frontiersin.org.
2. AAOS. Rickets. American Academy of Orthopedic Surgeons; 2021. https://orthoinfo.aaos.org.
3. MFMER. Rickets. Mayo Foundation for Medical Education and Research; 1998–2023. https://www.mayoclinic.org.

4. Gentile C, Chiarelli F. Rickets in children: an update. Biomedicines. 2021;9(7). https://www. ncbi.nlm.nih.gov.
5. Bikle DD. Vitamin D and the skin: physiology and pathophysiology. Rev Endocr Metab Disord. 2012;13(1). https://www.ncbi.nlm.nih.gov.
6. Mostafa WZ, Hegazy RH. Vitamin D and the skin: focus on a complex relationship: a review. J Adv Res. 2015;6(6). https://www.ncbi.nlm.nih.gov.
7. Yuen AWC, Jablonski NG. Vitamin D: in the evolution of skin color. Med Hypotheses. 2010;7(10). https://www.sciencedirect.com.
8. Dunn PM. Professor Armand Trousseau (1801-67) and the treatment of rickets. Arch Dis Childhood Fetal Neonatal Ed. 1999;80:F155–7. https://fn.bmj.com.
9. DeLuca HF. History of the discovery of vitamin D and its active metabolites. Bonekey Rep. 2014;3:479. https://www.ncbi.nlm.nih.gov.
10. Jones G. 100 Years of vitamin D: historical aspects of vitamin D. Endocr Connect. 2022;11(4). https://www.ncbi.nlm.nih.gov.
11. Holick MF. Resurrection of vitamin D deficiency and rickets. J Clin Invest. 2006;116(8). https://www.ncbi.nlm.nih.gov.
12. Rajakumar K, Thomas SB. Reemerging nutritional rickets: a historical perspective. Arch Pediatr Adolesc Med. 2005;159(4). https://jamanetwork.com.
13. CDC. Vitamin D. Centers for Disease Control and Prevention; 2021. https://www.cdc.gov.

Vitamin C Deficiency

14. CDC. Adult obesity facts. Centers for Disease Control and Prevention; 2022. https://www. cdc.gov.
15. Maxfield L, Crane JS. Vitamin C deficiency. NCBI Bookshelf: National Library of Medicine, National Institutes of Health; 2022. https://www.ncbi.nlm.nih.gov.
16. Johnson LE. Vitamin C deficiency (scurvy). Merck Manual: consumer edition. 2022. https:// www.merckmanuals.com.
17. Allan PK. Finding the cure for scurvy. Naval History Magaz. 2021;35(1). https://www.usni.org.
18. Price C. The age of scurvy. Science History Institute; 2017. https://www.sciencehistory.org.
19. Sutton G. Putrid gums and 'dead men's cloaths': James Lind Aboard the *Salisbury*. J R Soc Med. 2003;96(12). https://www.ncbi.nlm.nih.gov.
20. McCoy RM. Scurvy: the scourge of explorers. New World Exploration. 2014. https://www. newworldexploration.com.
21. Geber J, Murphy E. Scurvy in the Great Irish famine: evidence of vitamin C deficiency from mid-19th century skeletal population. Am J Phys Anthrop. 2012;148(4). https://www.ncbi. nlm.nih.gov.
22. Mayberry JA. A timeline of scurvy. Harvard Dash; 2004. https://dash.harvard.edu.
23. Lustrea J. Eat your (desiccated) vegetables. National Museum of Civil War Medicine; 2019. https://www.civilwarmed.org.
24. Carpenter KJ. The discovery of vitamin C. Ann Nutr Metab. 2012;61(3). https://pubmed.ncbi. nlm.nih.gov.
25. Dresen E, Lee Z-Y, Hill A, et al. History of scurvy and use of vitamin C in clinical illness: a narrative review. Nutr Clin Pract. 2023;38(1):46–54. https://pubmed.ncbi.nlm.nih.gov.
26. NIH: Vitamin C: fact sheet for health professionals. National Institutes of Health; 2021. https:// ods.od.nih.gov.

Chapter 9
Fungal Diseases

Abstract Fungal diseases are acquired by inhaling environmental fungal spores, contagious contact with infectious skin dermatophytes, or overgrowth of fungi normally inhabiting the skin or vagina. Some fungal infections can cause debilitating systemic infections and death. Others are nearly ubiquitous in nature and cause relatively minor infirmity. Some require aggressive medical management with prolonged administration of antifungal medications. Others can generally be dealt with using over-the-counter fungicidal creams.

The fungal diseases discussed in this chapter, along with their historical names and monikers, are: Coccidiomycosis (*Valley fever, Desert Rheumatism*); Dermatophytosis (*Ringworm*); and Candidiasis (*Vaginitis, Diaper Rash, Thrush*).

Coccidioidomycosis (*Valley Fever, Desert Rheumatism*)

Commonly referred to as "Valley fever," coccidioidomycosis generally presents as a pulmonary infection caused by inhaling dust particles containing spores of the *Coccidioides* fungus. Considered one of the most infectious fungal diseases, two different species are known to be causative agents: *Coccidioides immitis* and *C. posadasii* [1].

Coccidioides is a soil fungus, found almost exclusively in the Western Hemisphere in arid to semi-arid areas of the Southwestern United States, Mexico, and Central and South America. *C. immitis* is the species most common in the USA, most notably present in California's San Joaquin Valley, from which the moniker "Valley fever" is drawn [1, 2].

Many people exposed to the *Coccidioides* fungus never develop symptoms, others experience flu-like symptoms which may last several weeks or months. Symptoms may include fatigue, fever, night sweats, shortness of breath, headache,

J. A. Shaw, *Historical Diseases from a Modern Perspective*,
https://doi.org/10.1007/978-3-031-52346-5_9

Fig. 9.1 Rash (erythema nodosum) due to coccidioidomycosis. (Picture Source: https:// www.cdc.gov. CDC)

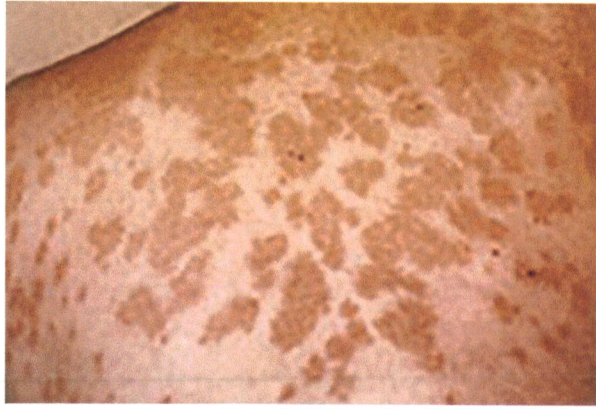

muscle aches, and joint pain. If accompanied by a nodular rash (erythema nodosum) (Fig. 9.1), the disease is sometimes referred to as "desert rheumatism" [2, 3].

Approximately 5–10% of infected persons develop serious long-term problems in their lungs, including chronic cough, pneumonia, hemoptysis, empyema, and hydropneumothorax. In approximately 1% of infected patients, the fungus spreads from the lungs to other parts of the body (disseminated coccidioidomycosis), including the skin, bones, joints, liver, kidneys, and brain. Infection of the brain and spinal cord (coccidioidal meningitis) may be life-threatening. Occasionally, skin infections may result from direct exposure to the fungus through cuts or abrasions [1–3].

Self-evidently, folks who live, work, and recreate in endemic areas, such as the San Joaquin Valley, are at most risk of contracting Valley fever. Among those, severe disease is most common in persons over 60 years of age, persons with weakened immune systems (diabetes, cancer, HIV/AIDS), pregnant women in the third trimester, and Blacks and Filipinos [3].

Pets, livestock, and wild animals are also susceptible to Valley fever the same way as humans, by breathing in spores of the *Coccidioides* fungus found in dirt and dust. As with humans, some animals may have no or mild illness, while others can experience severe disease and may die. Dogs are particularly susceptible, based on a propensity to dig in the dirt and sniff around rodent holes. Although principally affecting the lungs, an infected animal's symptoms will vary depending on how widespread the infection is and which organ systems are involved [4].

Valley fever is not contagious, with disease prophylaxis centered on avoiding breathing in large amounts of dust if living or recreating in an endemic area. Wearing N95 respirators, using indoor air filters, staying inside during dust storms, and avoiding gardening or other soil activities may all be helpful. Diagnosis is based on clinical presentation coupled with exposure likelihood, blood tests for *Coccidioides* antibodies or antigens, a chest X-ray or CT scan for characteristic lung imaging, and a lung biopsy for fungus culture. In severe/protracted cases, treatment with antifungal medications including fluconazole, itraconazole, or amphotericin B may be indicated [3].

****

According to the California Department of Public Health (CDPH), the number of Valley fever cases in California has markedly increased in recent years, with the number of reported cases tripling in the interval from 2014 to 2018. Between 7000 and 9000 California cases have been reported each year from 2018 to 2022, up from less than 1000 cases in 2000 [4].

Similar country-wide increases have been noted by the CDC, with 20,003 cases reported in 2019 (most commonly in persons living in Arizona and California), with tens of thousands of additional cases likely unreported or misdiagnosed [5]. The University of Arizona Valley Fever Center for Excellence estimates that Valley fever costs Arizona dog owners at least $60 million per year, entailing the diagnosis, treatment, and follow-up care of their infected dogs [6].

One of the probable reasons for the increased incidence of Valley fever is the protracted periods of drought in the Southwest in recent years, likely precipitated by climate change [7]. Self-evidently, drought-induced dust storms increase potential exposure to spore-laden dust. More specifically, it appears that a rainy winter following a period of drought creates the ideal conditions for the *Coccidioides* fungus to thrive and reproduce. Valley fever spores are able to survive in an inactive state during drought conditions that may be lethal to other types of soil microbes. A brief period of winter precipitation reactivates the spores, vastly increasing their soil numbers and apparent infectivity. During an ensuing dry period, the newly formed fungus-laden dust disseminates readily to exposed humans and animals, precipitating an outbreak of disease [4, 8].

Dermatophytosis (*Ringworm, Athlete's Foot, "Jock Itch"*)

Dermatophytosis, commonly referred to as "ringworm," is a fungal infection of skin caused by a large variety of dermatophytes (fungi), most commonly of the *Trichophyton*, *Microsporum*, or *Epidermophyton* type [9]. The "ringworm" moniker derives from the characteristic raised, red, itchy, circular rash that forms on the skin in the infected area (Fig. 9.2).

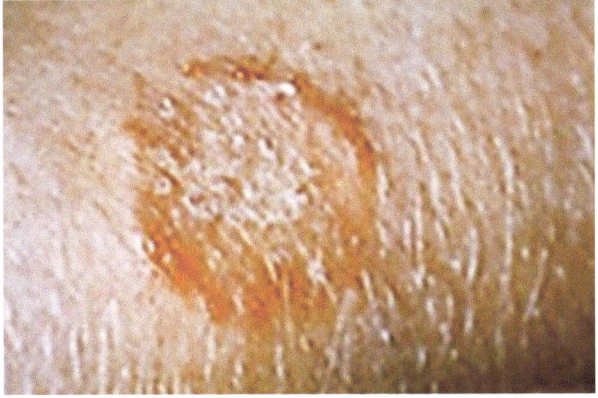

Fig. 9.2 Ringworm on the arm. (Picture Source: https://www.cdc. gov. CDC)

Ringworm is a very common and highly contagious infection, thought to affect 20–25% of the world's population at any given time [10]. Dermatophytes metabolize and subsist on keratin in the skin, hair, and nails and can spread from person-to-person through direct contact (e.g., contact sports) or via shared clothing, combs, or other personal items. They can also spread from pets or farm animals or from the environment, particularly from public showers or locker rooms where the skin fungi thrive [9–11].

Although recognized as an ancient affliction, fungal skin infections are largely overlooked in medical history because they rarely cause severe or life-threatening illness [12]. However, ringworm infections can cause intense social stigma, severe physical discomfort, and a decreased quality of life. When affecting different parts of the body, fungal skin infections commonly go by area-specific names [9, 13]:

- Arms or legs (tinea corporis)
- Feet (tinea pedis or *athlete's foot*)
- Groin (tinea cruris or *"jock itch"*)
- Scalp (tinea capitis)
- Beard (tinea barbae)
- Hands (tinea magnum)
- Nails (tinea unguium or onychomycosis)

Although ringworm of one form or another is nearly a ubiquitous affliction, those persons with a compromised immune system (HIV/AIDS, cancer, diabetes) are at greater risk of fungal skin infections, as are those who frequent public showers or locker rooms, participate in contact sports, wear tight clothing, sweat excessively, or are in close contact with animals [9, 10].

Prevention of infection centers on keeping the skin meticulously clean and dry, limiting the use of public locker rooms and showers, changing undergarments frequently, not sharing personal items or sports equipment, and avoiding contact with infected pets or farm animals. Diagnosis is based on clinical presentation coupled with microscopic examination or culture of skin scrapings [9, 10].

Most forms of ringworm can be successfully treated with non-prescription antifungal creams, such as clotrimazole or miconazole, applied to the skin for 2–4 weeks. Ringworm of the scalp (tinea capitis) (Fig. 9.3) generally requires prescription antifungal drugs, such as griseofulvin, ketoconazole, or fluconazole, taken by mouth for 1–3 months. Application of steroid creams to any ringworm infection is contraindicated and may make the infection worse [9].

****

Like so many other types of infections, the treatment of ringworm is currently compromised by the emergence of antimicrobial resistant organisms [9, 14]. According to the CDC, contributing factors include the overuse of non-prescription topical antifungal creams, inappropriate use of steroid creams, inappropriate prescription of antifungal medications, and inadequate adherence to a prescribed regimen of antifungal drugs [9]. Global travel and migration transport resistant organisms around the world, exacerbating the problem.

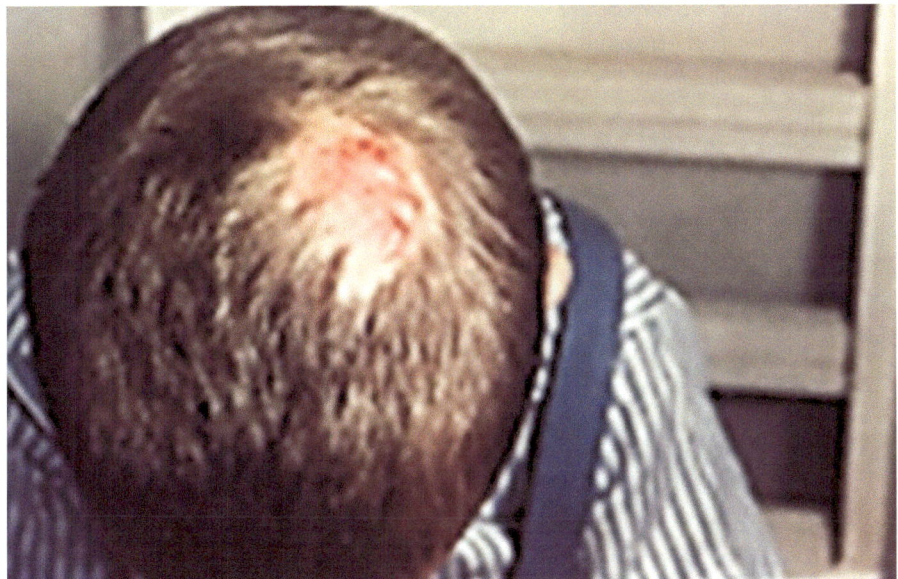

Fig. 9.3 Ringworm on the scalp. (Picture Source: https://www.cdc.gov. CDC)

N.B.
The reader is referred to the informative and graphic web page produced by the American Academy of Dermatology [13] *for photographs of ringworm affecting different body areas.*

Candidiasis (*Vaginitis, Diaper Rash, Thrush*)

Candidiasis is an infection caused by overgrowth of a yeast fungus called *Candida*. Normally, a commensal organism of the skin, gastrointestinal tract, and vagina, *Candida* species (commonly *C. albicans*) can multiply and cause an infection if the inhibitory balance of native healthy bacteria is altered—typically following a course of antibiotics, among other factors—allowing unchecked overgrowth of the yeast.

Three common types of candidiasis, with their colloquial names, are generally recognized [15, 16]:

1. *Vaginal candidiasis (Vaginitis)*: A common infection, often following a course of antibiotics, during pregnancy, or in association with diabetes or other immune disorders, resulting in vaginal discharge, burning, itching, and discomfort during intercourse or when urinating.
2. *Cutaneous candidiasis (Diaper Rash)*: A common infection of the skin resulting in an itchy, raised, red, rash, generally in moist intertriginous areas (skin folds) such as under the breasts, axilla, abdomen, groin, or on the buttocks under a wet diaper.

Fig. 9.4 White patchy lesions of oral candidiasis (thrush). (Picture Source: https://phil.cdc.gov. CDC: Public Health Image Library)

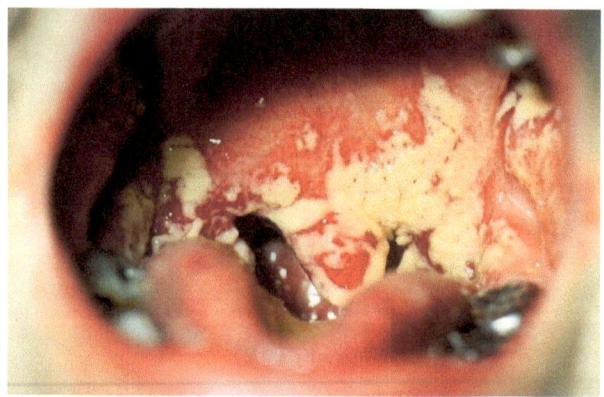

3. *Oral candidiasis* (*Thrush*): An infection of the mouth and throat, with resultant white patches on the inner cheeks, tongue, roof of mouth and throat, often associated with pain when eating or swallowing, loss of taste, and a cotton-like sensation in the mouth (Fig. 9.4).

Candida granuloma is a rare and refractory cutaneous candidiasis usually reported in immunocompromised patients [17]. Invasive candidiasis is a serious fungal infection, most commonly involving the bloodstream (candidemia), but may also involve the heart (endocarditis), brain (meningitis), and other organ systems [18]. Most often occurring in immunocompromised patients, the associated in-hospital mortality of invasive candidiasis is approximately 30% [18].

Factors disrupting the normal balance of bacteria and yeast and triggering the more common types of candidiasis include taking antibiotics, steroids, oral contraceptives, and medicines that cause dry mouth. Additionally, a diet in refined carbohydrates, uncontrolled diabetes (or other immunocompromising diseases), stress, and hormonal changes of pregnancy are recognized triggering factors [15, 16].

The diagnosis of candidiasis is principally based on clinical presentation, but may involve swabbing the infected area for microscopic examination and culture. Invasive candidiasis is defined by blood culture. Candidiasis is not conventionally contagious but direct contact with skin or oral lesions (transfer of saliva) may alter the balance of bacteria and yeast and cause a transferred infection.

Treatment of the three common *Candida* infections usually involves application of non-prescription antifungal medications, including clotrimazole, miconazole, or nystatin, as a cream, suppository, lozenge, pill, or liquid depending on the infection location (skin, vagina, mouth), with expectation of a rapid resolution of the infection. For severe infections, fluconazole or other antifungal drugs may be prescribed as an oral or intravenous medication and may necessitate a protracted therapeutic course [15–18].

Unfortunately, as noted in the discussions of treatment in virtually every other disease section, treatment of *Candida* infections has become increasingly compromised by the emergence of antimicrobial resistance [19].

References

Coccidioidomycosis

1. Garcia SCG, Alanis JCS, Flores MG, et al. Coccidioidomycosis and the skin: a comprehensive review. An Bras Dermatol. 2015;90(5):610. https://www.ncbi.nlm.nih.gov.
2. CDC. Valley fever (Coccidioidomycosis). Centers for Disease Control and Prevention; 2020. https://www.cdc.gov.
3. Cleveland Clinic. Valley fever (Coccidioidomycosis). Cleveland Clinic; 2022. https://my.clevelandclinic.org.
4. CDPH. Valley fever is on the rise in California. California Department of Public Health; 2023. https://www.cdph.ca.gov.
5. CDC. Valley fever (Coccidioidomycosis) statistics. Centers for Disease Control and Prevention; 2020. https://www.cdc.gov.
6. VFCE. Valley fever in dogs. The University of Arizona College of Medicine Valley Fever Center for Excellence; 2021. https://vfce.arizona.edu.
7. American Lung Association. How climate change has led to an increase in valley fever. 2017. https://www.lung.org.
8. Head JR, Sondermeyer-Cooksey G, Heaney AK, et al. Effects of precipitation, heat, and drought on incidence and expansion of coccidioidomycosis in western USA: a longitudinal surveillance study. Lancet Planet Earth. 2022;6(10):e793–803. https://www.ncbi.nlm.nih.gov.

Dermatophytosis

9. CDC. Ringworm. Centers for Disease Control and Prevention; 2021. https://www.cdc.gov.
10. Cleveland Clinic. Ringworm. Cleveland Clinic; 2022. https://my.clevelandvlinc.org.
11. Hainer BL. Dermatophyte infections. Am Fam Physician. 2003;67(1):101–8. https://www.aafp.org.
12. Worboys HA, Basingstoke M. Fungal diseases in Britain and the United States 1850-2000: mycoses and modernity. NCBI Bookshelf: National Library of Medicine, National Institutes of Health; 2013. https://www.ncbi.nlm.nih.gov.
13. AAD. Ringworm: signs and symptoms. American Academy of Dermatology Association; 2023. https://www.aad.org.
14. Hay RJ. The spread of resistant tinea and the ingredients of a perfect storm. Dermatology. 2022;238(1):80–1. https://karger.com.

Candidiasis

15. CDC. Fungal diseases: candidiasis. Centers for Disease Control and Prevention; 2022. https://www.cdc.gov.
16. Cleveland Clinic. Candidiasis. Cleveland Clinic; 2022. https://my.clevelandclinic.org.
17. Yang H, Xu X, Ran X, et al. Successful treatment of refractory candidal granuloma by itraconazole and terbinafine in combination with hyperthermia and cryotherapy. Dermatol Ther. 2020;10(4):847–53. https://www.ncbi.nlm.nih.gov.
18. CDC. Fungal diseases: information for healthcare professionals about invasive candidiasis. Centers for Disease Control and Prevention; 2022. https://www.cdc.gov.
19. CDC. Fungal diseases: antimicrobial resistance in *Candida*. Centers for Disease Control and Prevention; 2022. https://www.cdc.gov.

Chapter 10
Soil-Related Bacterial Diseases

Abstract Soil-related bacterial infections are caused by soil contamination of open wounds, or by inhalation, ingestion, or skin contact with soil-indigenous bacterial spores. Although uncommon in number, the infections caused by the toxin-producing soil bacteria discussed in this chapter are remarkably virulent and often cause death. Of particular concern is the potential use of anthrax spores as an agent of bioterrorism.

The soil-related bacterial diseases discussed in this chapter, along with their historical names and monikers, are: Tetanus (*Lockjaw*); Anthrax (*Woolsorter's Disease, Malignant Pustule*); and Clostridial Myonecrosis (*Gas Gangrene*).

Tetanus (*Lockjaw*)

Like soil-borne fungi, many types of indigenous soil bacteria can cause serious infections in humans, including wound, skin, gastrointestinal and pulmonary diseases [1].

Of the many soil-related bacterial diseases, tetanus is perhaps the most familiar by name to most Americans, with an awareness based on its ubiquitous childhood vaccination protocol and its recommended 10-year-interval booster shots, as well as its horrifyingly descriptive "lockjaw" moniker.

Tetanus is caused by the spore-forming, gram-positive, rod-shaped, obligate anaerobic bacterium, *Clostridium tetani* (Fig. 10.1). As with diphtheria and pertussis, it is an exotoxin (*tetanospasmin*) produced by the bacterium that is the principal cause of tetanus symptoms, not the bacteria itself. Referred to as tetanus toxin, *tetanospasmin* is one of the most potent neurotoxins known [2, 3].

The spores produced by the tetanus bacterium are ubiquitously distributed in the environment, especially organic-rich soil, and are highly resistant to heat,

J. A. Shaw, *Historical Diseases from a Modern Perspective*,
https://doi.org/10.1007/978-3-031-52346-5_10

Fig. 10.1 Lantern slide
showing rod-shaped
C. tetani bacteria with
rounded spore protrusions
at one end. Circa early
1900s. (Picture Source:
https://www.si.edu. The
City of New York Dept. of
Health)

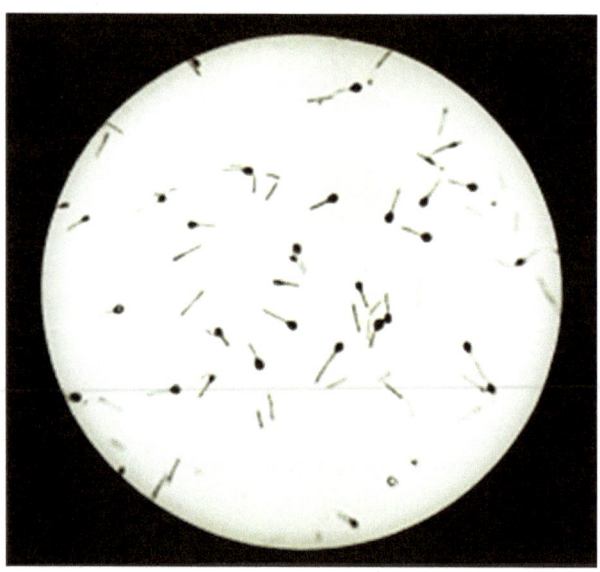

desiccation and disinfectants. Additionally, the spores are commonly present in the intestines and feces of horses, sheep, cattle and other animals, which can further contaminate manure-enriched soil.

When tetanus spores are introduced into the body—most notably in the anaerobic environment created by a skin puncture wound (often by a dirty nail)—they germinate into active bacteria, releasing the potent tetanospasmin neurotoxin, causing the clinical manifestations of tetanus. The toxin blocks inhibitory neurotransmitters, leading to unopposed muscle contraction and spasm [2–4].

Four different forms of tetanus are commonly recognized [2, 4, 5]. Generalized tetanus (80% of reported cases) is initially characterized by trismus (spasm of the jaw muscles, referred to as "lockjaw"), generally followed by nuchal (neck muscle) rigidly, dysphagia (difficulty swallowing), and rigidity of abdominal muscles. As the disease progresses, generalized muscle rigidly, backward arching of the head, neck and spine (*opisthotonos*), and intermittent spasms may ensue, sometimes with enough force to cause fractures (Fig. 10.2). Contraction of facial muscles may produce a sneering grin, referred to as *risus sardonicus*. Fever, sweating, elevated blood pressure, and tachycardia are common. Respiratory failure and cardiac arrest are life-threatening complications. Spasms can continue for 3–4 weeks, and full recovery may take months.

In rare cases, persons may be afflicted with localized tetanus where muscle contractions are limited to the anatomic area of the tetanus bacteria inoculation. Contractions may last for weeks and may progress into generalized tetanus, albeit generally milder.

Cranial nerve involvement following a head injury or middle ear infection (otitis media) is a rare form of tetanus, referred to as cephalic tetanus.

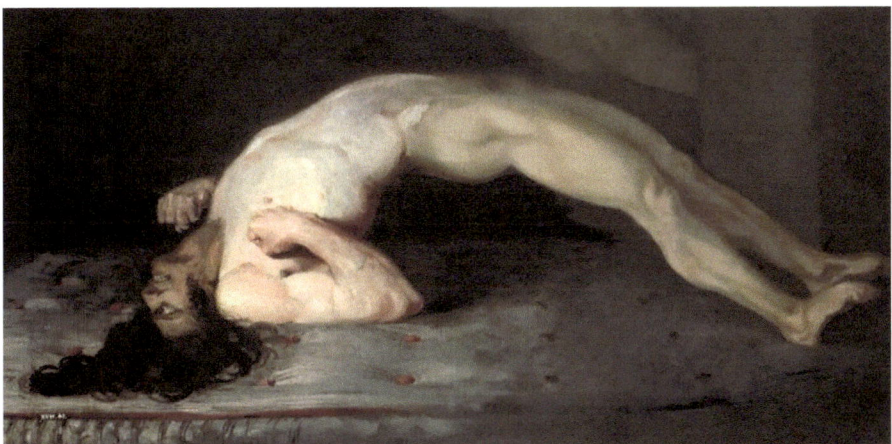

Fig. 10.2 Opisthotonos in a patient suffering from tetanus. "*Tetanus Following Gunshot Wounds*". Artist: Sir Charles Bell, Circa 1809. (Picture Source: https://commons.wikimedia.org)

Fig. 10.3 Neonatal tetanus opisthotonos. (Picture Source: https://phil.cdc. gov. CDC: Public Health Image Library)

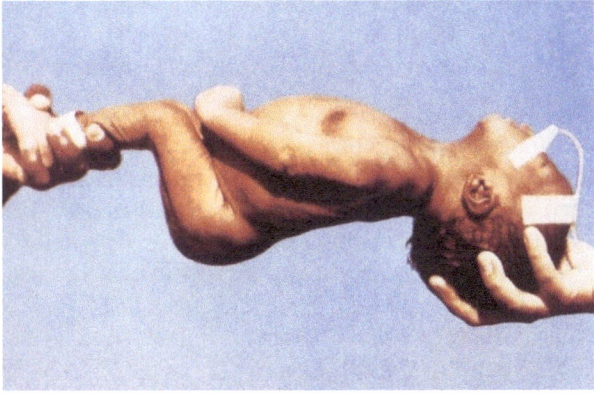

Neonatal tetanus (*tetanus neonatorum*) occurs in newborn infants and is a major cause of infant mortality in third-world countries. It is a form of generalized tetanus that generally follows an infection of the umbilical cord stump—most frequently when the cord is cut with unsterile instruments—in an infant without passive immunity due to the lack of maternal immunization (Fig. 10.3).

****

Tetanus spores can enter the body through any break in the skin, but most commonly through puncture wounds, wounds contaminated by dirt and feces, crush injuries, burns, compound fractures, and contaminated needle (heroin) sticks. The incubation period between exposure and clinical illness ranges from 3 to 21 days (average 8 days), but symptoms/signs are most commonly evident within 14 days [6].

Tetanus is diagnosed entirely on the clinical presentation of trismus, dysphagia, muscle rigidity, and spasms and does not require laboratory confirmation [4]. The WHO clinical criteria for diagnosis of neonatal tetanus are based on an infant's loss of his or her preexisting ability to suckle and cry in the interval between 3 and 28 days of life, and exhibits an associated rigidity or spasms during the same interval. The diagnosis of non-neonatal tetanus is based on spasms of facial muscles (lockjaw) or other painful muscular contractions, generally in conjunction with a history of injury or a wound (which in some cases may not be recognized or appreciated). Wound culture is only marginally helpful in that it is fraught with false positives and false negatives [2, 7].

Treatment of tetanus is a hospital-based medical emergency and is centered on [2, 4, 5, 7]:

- Aggressive wound debridement to remove necrotic tissue and create an open-wound aerobic environment.
- Immediate administration of human tetanus immune globulin (TIG) to neutralize unbound neuron tetanus toxin.
- Drugs to control muscle spasms.
- Antibiotics to kill remaining toxin-producing *C. tetani* bacteria.
- Active immunization with tetanus toxoid.
- Ventilation support, as needed.
- Treatment of nosocomial infections, pressure sores, pulmonary emboli, and other secondary complications.

Historically, tetanus disease progression resulted in death in approximately 85% of those infected [3]. With current medical management the death rate is between 10% and 20% [6]. WHO data [7] indicates that approximately 25,000 newborns died worldwide from neonatal tetanus in 2018, a mortality statistic that has decreased by 97% since 1998, principally through a scaled-up global immunization initiative with tetanus-toxoid-containing vaccines (TTCV). Recovery from an active infection does not result in life-long immunity. A person with active disease is not contagious.

****

Although clinical descriptions of tetanus date to the 5th century BCE, it was not until 1884 that tetanus was produced in animals with an injection of pus from a fatal human tetanus case. The same year, a definitive link to soil contamination of wounds as the primary source of the disease was established by German physician Arthur Nicolaier (1862–1942) by injecting mice with soil inoculums [8, 9].

During the 1890s, the combined efforts of Japanese physician Shibasaburo Kitasato (1853–1931), 1901 German Nobel laureate Emil von Behring (1845–1917), and French veterinarian and microbiologist Edmond Nocard (1850–1903) demonstrated that tetanus antitoxin had both protective and immunizing efficacy against tetanus [3, 9, 10].

Antitoxins were initially developed by injecting horses with increasing doses of tetanus toxin, allowing their immune systems to generate antitoxins (antibodies) to

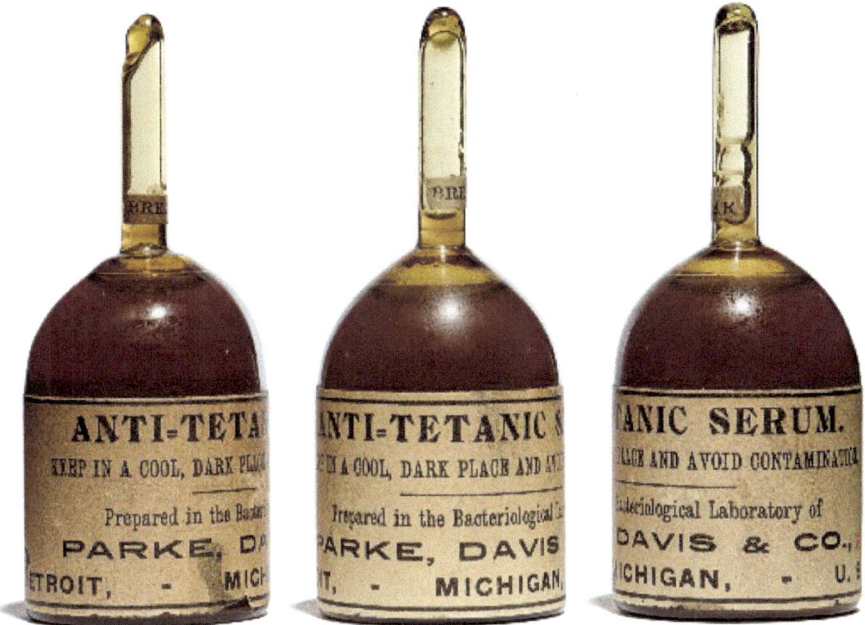

Fig. 10.4 Anti-tetanic horse serum. Circa 1898. Parke, Davis & Co. (Picture Source: https://www.si.edu. Smithsonian Institution)

neutralize the toxins (Fig. 10.4).[1] Horse serum antitoxin was used extensively in WWI in a desperate attempt to avoid tetanus' high fatality rate, most commonly following war wounds contaminated by soil or by soil-covered shrapnel driven deep into tissue. Many soldiers developed allergic reactions ("serum sickness") to the horse serum, but horse serum antitoxin is credited with saving hundreds of thousands of lives in WWI [3, 8].

Today, tetanus immune globulin is derived from the plasma of human volunteers who have been fully immunized against tetanus. Produced by Grifols Therapeutics, Inc., the HyperTet® globulin is the only approved product for unvaccinated tetanus prophylaxis and therapeutic use in the USA at this time [11].

In the 1920s, a method of inactivating tetanus toxin with formaldehyde was developed, leading to the development of the tetanus toxoid vaccine in 1924, first widely used during WWII. In the late 1940s tetanus toxoid vaccines were introduced into routine childhood vaccination protocols and in 1948 the vaccine was produced in combination with the diphtheria toxoid and the pertussis vaccine, forming the ubiquitous DPT vaccine.

---

[1] The reader is referred to the Smithsonian Institution's web page https://www.si.edu/spotlight/antibody-initiative/battling-tetanus for a fascinating pictorial review of early tetanus toxin and toxoid vaccinations.

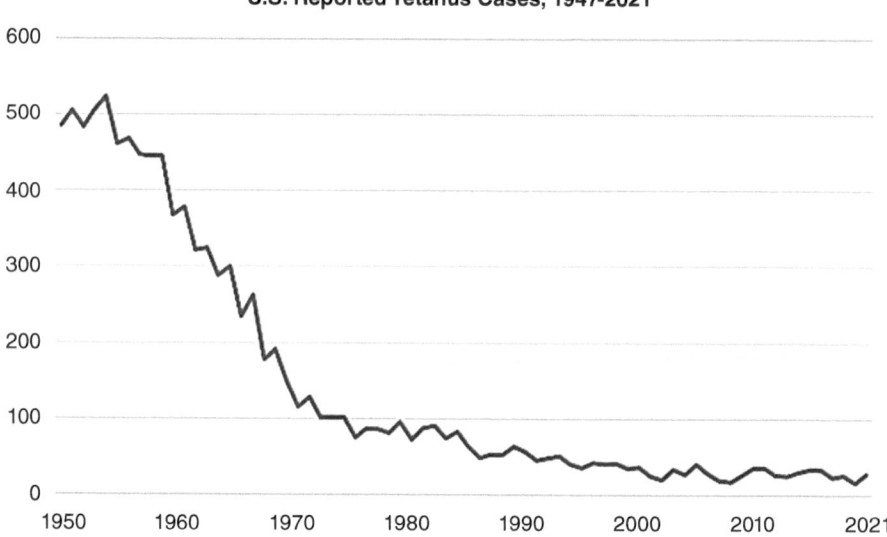

Fig. 10.5 CDC data regarding reported tetanus cases (1947–2021). (Picture Source: https://www. cdc.gov. CDC)

With routine childhood vaccination, the incidence of tetanus in the USA declined steadily (Fig. 10.5). In the 1940s there were between 500 and 600 cases reported annually. By the mid-1970s the case incidence had dropped to about 50–100 cases/ year. Between 2009 and 2018 the case numbers further dropped to an average of 29 per year (297 cases total) with 19 deaths, all in patients over 55 years of age [2, 9].

According to the CDC, sporadic tetanus cases continue to date, principally in adults who have never received a tetanus vaccination or who have neglected to update their initial vaccination with periodic 10-year booster shots [6].

Routine childhood immunization against tetanus is currently recommended in the USA and throughout most of the world. Tetanus toxoid is generally administered in combination with diphtheria toxoid and acellular pertussis vaccine (DTaP) in various dose regimens depending on the patient's age and history of prior immunizations.

Recent statistics indicate that vaccination compliance within the States is high among children (93.3%) but lower among adults (63.4%) [2]. The WHO reports that 84% of infants worldwide were vaccinated with three doses of diphtheria-tetanus-pertussis (DTP) containing vaccines in 2022 [7].

Anthrax (*Woolsorter's Disease, Malignant Pustule*)

Without question, the word that comes to mind with the mention of anthrax is not one of its historical nicknames, horrific as they may sound. The word is BIOTERRORISM!

Anthrax is a rare infectious disease of animals and humans caused by the gram-positive, spore-forming bacterium, *Bacillus anthracis.* Anthrax bacteria reside in environmental soil, producing dormant spores that are resistant to extremes of temperature, desiccation, radiation, and disinfectants and can survive for protracted periods of time. An ancient disease, the bacterium was first identified in the 1800s and formed the experimental basis for Kock's postulates (1877), discussed in the introductory chapter [12, 13].

Domestic or wild grazing animals can become infected when they breathe in or ingest environmental spores. Although an uncommon affliction in the developed world, humans historically contracted the disease by eating the meat or handling the wool, hair, hides, bone or carcasses of infected animals—likely accounting for the moniker "Woolsorter's disease." It is also possible for people to become infected directly, by inhalation of environmental spores, eating or drinking spore-contaminated food or water, or by entry of spore-containing soil into cuts or scrapes [12, 13].

When anthrax spores enter the body, they germinate into active bacteria which release a tripartite exotoxin causing symptomatic disease, much like the tetanus toxin discussed in the previous section. Simplistically stated, anthrax toxins hijack the immune system, allowing proliferation and spread of bacteria and in severe cases leading to death of the host [14].

There are four recognized types of anthrax infections, each with different presentations. Under most circumstances, anthrax is not a communicable disease. Symptoms typically develop within 6 days of exposure, with the exception of inhalation anthrax where symptomatic disease may take more than 6 weeks to present [12, 15, 16].

Cutaneous anthrax results from the entry of anthrax spores through the skin, typically via a cut or abrasion. Historically most common among workers in the animal hair industry, cutaneous anthrax is the mildest form of the disease, being seldom fatal. The initial infection results in a raised itchy bump that develops into a painless sore with a black center (the "malignant pustule") over time (Fig. 10.6). In a majority of cases the bacilli remain within the sore, but occasionally may spread

Fig. 10.6 Anthrax cutaneous skin lesion ("malignant pustule"). (Picture Source: https://phil.cdc.gov. CDC: Public Health Image Library)

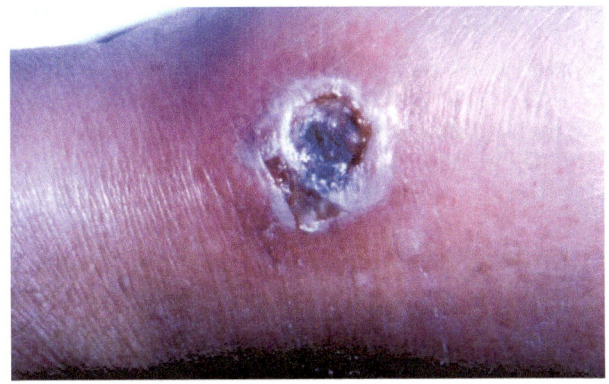

to the nearest lymph node and in rare cases to the bloodstream causing internal bleeding, meningitis, and fatal septicemia. Flu-like symptoms of fever and head-ache may accompany the localized infection [12, 15].

Gastrointestinal anthrax results from ingestion of undercooked meat from an animal infected with anthrax. Infection may involve the oropharyngeal area as well as the more common gastrointestinal tract, with a symptom complex including fever, nausea and vomiting, sore throat, and severe bloody diarrhea. Systemic spread of bacteria to the bloodstream can result in death in 25–60% of persons afflicted with this form of the disease, according to CDC estimates [12, 15].

The deadliest form of the disease is inhalation anthrax, resulting from breathing in anthrax spores. Aerosolized spores released during the processing of animal hides, wool or hair was the principal mode of infection from a historical perspective. Aerosolized spores released into the atmosphere during a bioterrorist attack is the mode of infection of most concern at the present time [12, 15].

Initial symptoms of inhalation anthrax resemble a common cold, including fever, chills, body ache, and cough. Progression of the disease results in chest pain, short-ness of breath, confusion, dizziness, drenching sweats, and extreme fatigue. Mortality rates have varied over time, ranging from 85% in historical cases to 45% in the 2001 U.S. bioterrorism attack, despite aggressive antibiotic therapy and mod-ern respiratory support [12, 15].

A new type of anthrax was recently identified (2010) in Europe among heroin drug users—referred to as injection anthrax. The heroin injections in the reported cases resulted in swelling and infection in deep layers of tissue, without the raised sore with a black center characteristic of cutaneous anthrax. The infective etiology was positively identified in the affected patients by direct culture of the anthrax organism or by polymerase chain reaction (PCR)—the presumptive source being a spore-contaminated heroin supply. Massive edema, necrotizing fasciitis, shock, multiple organ failure, and meningitis were reported in some cases, with death in around 30% of the affected patients [15, 17].

****

Although rare in the USA, anthrax is still common in the developing world, with most human cases resulting from exposure to infected animals or their meat, fur, or hides. In 1937 Italian immunologist Max Sterne (1905–1995) developed a live spore vaccine for animals [18]. Coupled with improvements in animal product pro-cessing, the routine vaccination of farm animals precipitously dropped the number of anthrax cases in humans. Notably, there were only 18 cases of inhalation anthrax during the entire twentieth century in the USA, according to CDC data [13].

The diagnosis of anthrax is made by clinical presentation in association with an animal exposure history, and confirmed by isolating the anthrax bacillus from blood, skin lesions, stool, spinal fluid or respiratory secretions (Fig. 10.7). A chest X-ray or CT scan may be helpful in diagnosing inhalation anthrax and antibody and polymerase chain reaction (PCR) tests may also be of diagnostic help in some cases [12, 19].

Treatment of anthrax is centered on antibiotic and antitoxin administration in addition to supportive care as needed. Antibiotics such as ciprofloxacin,

Fig. 10.7 Anthrax bacteria growing on culture medium. (Picture Source: https://phil.cdc.gov. CDC: Public Health Image Library)

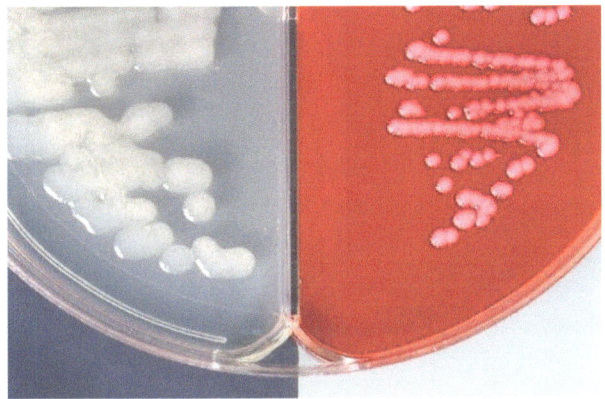

doxycycline, and levofloxacin have replaced penicillin as the antibiotic of choice for the treatment of anthrax and are frequently used in combination to kill the anthrax bacteria. Antitoxins (*Raxibacumab* and *Obiltoxaximab*) are approved for use in inhalation anthrax cases. They bind to the protective antigen (PA) of *Bacillus anthracis*, limiting its destructive effects by blocking entry of the toxin into cells. Human immune globulin (*Anthrasil*) is also available and is also approved for treatment of inhalation anthrax in adult and pediatric patients when used in combination with antibiotic therapy [19–21].

The first successful anthrax vaccine for use in humans was developed in the 1950s. Initially tested in goat hair millworkers, the vaccine demonstrated an efficacy of 92.5% in preventing cutaneous anthrax [13]. The vaccine was updated in 1970, and two similar vaccines (*BioThrax* and *Cyfendus*) are currently FDA approved and available for use in persons 18–65 years of age, following suspected or confirmed exposure to the *Bacillus anthracis* bacterium, when used in association with appropriate antibiotics. BioThrax is also approved for prophylactic protection in persons at high risk for exposure to the Anthrax bacillus, including research personnel working with the anthrax bacterium, some animal workers and veterinarians, and some members of the military. Additionally, vaccines have been purchased by the federal government and stockpiled in the Strategic National Stockpile for post-exposure prophylaxis in the event of a bioterrorist attack [12, 21–23].

****

The anthrax bacterium has several characteristics that make it ideally suited for use as a biological weapon.[2] Being a soil-indigenous species, *Bacillus anthracis* is widely available and easily accessible and is readily and inexpensively cultured in small and easily concealed laboratory settings. The spores are small enough to

---

[2] The history of biological weapons development and the international treaties designed to control their use is a fascinating subject, but beyond the scope of this book. A concise summary, specifically related to the use of anthrax, is available at the CDC website https://www.cdc.gov/anthrax/basics/anthrax-history.html in the section labeled Anthrax Used as a Biological Weapon.

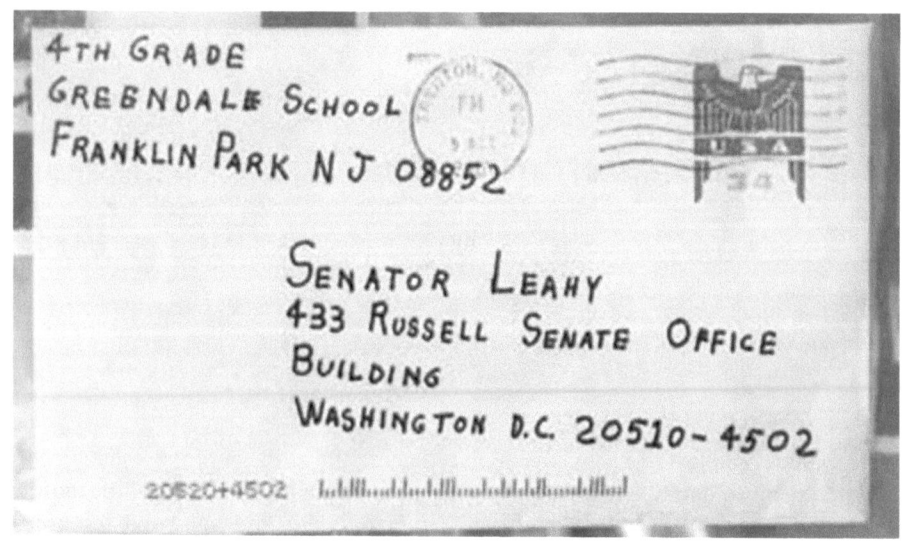

Fig. 10.8 Letter containing anthrax spores sent to Senator Leahy. (Picture Source: https://archives. fbi.gov/archives/about-us/history/famous-cases/anthrax-amerithrax/the-envelopes. FBI)

lodge readily in human lungs and have a short incubation period before germinating into viable bacteria, producing the deadly anthrax toxin. Moreover, they are highly resistant to ultraviolet light and can be readily prepared and distributed as a powder or a liquid, allowing use in a variety of weapon delivery systems [13, 16, 24].

Soon after the 9/11 terrorist attacks on the World Trade Center and Pentagon, letters laced with anthrax spores were mailed to the offices of U.S. Senators Leahy and Daschle and to various news broadcasters and outlets along the East Coast, postmarked September 18, and October 9, 2001 (Fig. 10.8).

The letter envelopes contained a very sophisticated "weapons-grade" preparation of anthrax spores, suggesting a governmental laboratory source, allowing the spores to float freely in the air, contaminating the postal facilities where they were processed, as well as the offices and buildings where they were opened. The letters all contained various versions of the cryptic message stating: *This is next; Take penicillin now; Death to America; Death to Israel; Allah is great.*[3]

There were 11 confirmed cases of inhalation anthrax and 11 confirmed cases of cutaneous anthrax resulting from this terrorist attack. Of the 22 persons afflicted, 5 died, all from cases of inhalation anthrax. In total, 43 persons tested positive for anthrax exposure and an estimated 10,000 persons were possibly exposed to one degree or another.

---

[3] The reader is referred to the informative FBI web page https://www.fbi.gov/history/famous-cases/ amerithrax-or-anthrax-investigation for details of the 2001 anthrax terrorist investigation, termed *Amerithrax.*

The FBI conducted an exhaustive 7-year investigation into the person or persons responsible for this act of terror. Laboratory/genetic analysis of the spores determined they were from the Ames strain—more specifically the RMR-1029 batch—which was traced to the United States Army Medical Research Institute of Infectious Diseases, Fort Detrick, Maryland. Research microbiologist Dr. Bruce Ivins was suspected of the crime, but took his own life before charges were formally filed. Following Ivins' suicide, the case investigation was concluded on February 19, 2010, without a complete understanding of the motive involved.

Of note, the Biological Weapons Convention treaty of 1972 [25], signed by the USA and 100 other nations, states in Article 1 that all parties under the Convention are:

Never to develop, produce, stockpile, or otherwise acquire or retain: (1) biological agents or toxins of types and in quantities that have no justification for peaceful uses; and (2) weapons, equipment, or means of delivery designed to use such agents or toxins for hostile purposes.

Clostridial Myonecrosis (*Gas Gangrene*)

Synonymous with the medical term *clostridial myonecrosis*, "gas gangrene" is the commonly used name depicting the horrific, often lethal infection of muscle and other soft tissues caused by *Clostridium* bacteria species, most commonly *C. perfringens* (Fig. 10.9).

Clostridium bacteria are toxin producing, anaerobic, spore-forming, gram-positive bacilli, ubiquitously found in soil and dust, but also commonly inhabiting the GI tract and female genital tract in humans. Classically associated with war

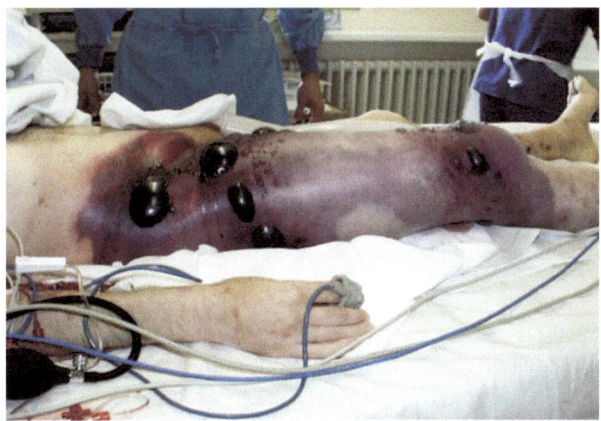

Fig. 10.9 Gas gangrene of the right leg and pelvis. License: Creative Commons Attribution 2.0 Generic (https://creativecommons.org/licenses/by/2.0/deed.en). (Picture Source: https://en.wikipedia.org. Engelbert Schröpfer, Stephan Rauthe and Thomas Meyer. Diagnosis and misdiagnosis of necrotizing soft tissue infections: three case reports. Cases J 2008, 1:252)

wounds, gas gangrene complicated many injuries during the American Civil War and 6% of open fractures and 1% of all open wounds suffered by U.S. soldiers in WWI [26]. With the advent of antibiotics and advancements in medical and surgical care, the incidence of gas gangrene infections progressively decreased during ensuing wars, becoming vanishingly small (0.002%) at the time of the Vietnam War [26].

Albeit relatively rare in the civilian population, gas gangrene is associated with abdominal wounds, open-wound extremity injuries and fractures, gunshot and knife wounds, crush injuries, and farm accidents, but is also a recognized complication of abdominal surgery and may present seemingly spontaneously with leakage of bacteria from the gut into the bloodstream in cases of colon cancer, diverticulitis, and other abdominal lesions [26–29].

The virulence of clostridial organisms depends on the production and release of exotoxins, *C. perfringens* being the most lethal with the production of multiple known toxins—the most destructive being the alpha-toxin which is a phospholipase (lecithinase) that damages cell membranes and triggers platelet aggregation, thrombosis of blood vessels and histamine release. Other toxins produced by *C. perfringens* cause direct vascular injury and lysis of leukocytes (white cells), inhibiting the host response to the infection. Additionally, toxin collagenases break down connective tissue, allowing spread of the infection across tissue planes [26, 28].

Typically, the incubation period for gas gangrene is short (<24 h), with rapidly multiplying organisms spewing out locally and systemically injurious toxins within hours of inoculation. Gas production likely results from the fermentation of glucose, with resultant gas dissection within muscles and along fascial planes, facilitating the spread of infection. Mortality figures hover around 25–30% with prompt medical care, but approach 100% in spontaneous cases and in cases where treatment is delayed [26, 28].

Necrotizing fasciitis may present in a similar fashion to gas gangrene, in that both types of infection destroy tissue and may be fatal. The principal distinction is the tissue types involved and the different infecting organisms. Necrotizing fasciitis tracks along fascial planes and destroys subcutaneous fat. Gas gangrene mainly destroys muscle tissue, blood cells, and blood vessels, as noted above. Whereas gas gangrene is typically caused by *C. perfringens*, necrotizing fasciitis is usually caused by group A *Streptococcus* or *Staphylococcus aureus* [30].

Tissue necrosis due to vascular injury or disease and the resultant interruption of oxygenated blood supply is often referred to as "dry gangrene." Dry gangrene does not have an infectious etiology, although secondary infections may occur.

****

Symptoms and signs of gas gangrene include rapid onset of pain and swelling following an injury resulting from a dirty, open wound. The skin color around the contaminated wound typically progresses from a bronze hue to an overt black and blue color with skin blebs and hemorrhagic bullae. The wound may have a foul, sweet or mousy odor and exhibit crepitus due to gas production. Pain and tenderness are frequently disproportionately severe in comparison to the wound appearance.

Fever, tachycardia, hypotension, renal failure, disseminated intravascular coagulation (DIC), acute respiratory distress, altered mental status, and a feeling of impending doom are common. Shock and death commonly follow without emergent care. Spontaneous-onset (gastrointestinal) cases present similarly, but without an external wound [26, 30]

The diagnosis of gas gangrene is principally based on clinical presentation. Imaging studies classically show gas infiltrates within muscle tissue (Fig. 10.10). Gram stains of exudate or infected tissue typically show gram-positive clostridia bacilli, but often with paradoxically few accompanying white cells. Tissue cultures are generally positive for the infecting organism and help direct antibiotic therapy based on drug sensitivity testing. Metabolic abnormalities (acidosis and renal failure) are commonly evident on routine blood chemistry profiles [26, 28–30].

Treatment of gas gangrene is focused on early and aggressive surgical debridement of infected tissue, frequently involving amputation of limbs in cases of extremity infections. Immediate empirical initiation of broad-spectrum antibiotics is imperative, pending culture sensitivity results. Historically, penicillin G was the antibiotic of choice for *C. perfringens*, now generally administered in combination with clindamycin [26, 28]. The use of hyperbaric oxygen following surgical debridement is controversial [26] but reduces mortality significantly according to some studies [28]. Ventilatory and hemodynamic support are integral parts of the therapeutic regimens of all critically ill patients, including patients suffering from gas gangrene.

Fig. 10.10 X-ray showing gas in tissue planes in a patient with gas gangrene. Created by user شهاب on Wiki Commons. License: Creative Commons Attribution-Share Alike 4.0, https://creativecommons.org/licenses/by-sa/4.0/. (Picture Source: https://www.ncbi.nlm.nih.gov)

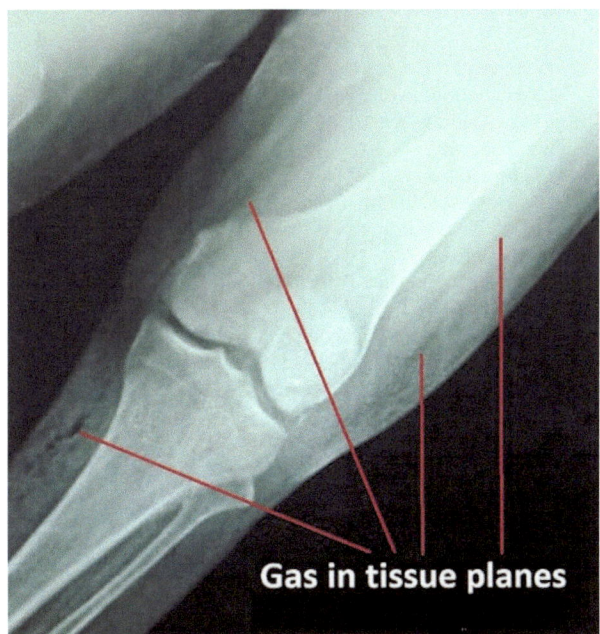

Gas in tissue planes

References

Tetanus

1. Baumgardner DJ. Soil-related bacterial and fungal infections. JABFM. 2012;25(5):734–44. https://www.jabfm.org.
2. Tiwari TSP, Moro PL, Acosta AM. Epidemiology and prevention of vaccine-preventable diseases: tetanus. In: "The Pink Book". 14th ed. Centers for Disease Control and Prevention; 2021. https://www.cdc.gov.
3. Smithsonian Institution. Antibody initiative: battling tetanus. Smithsonian Institution; Undated. https://www.si.edu.
4. Hinfey PB, Brusch JL. editors. Tetanus. Medscape. 2023. https://emedicine.medscape.com.
5. Shahade A, De Jesus O. Opisthotonos. In: StatPearls. New York: National Institutes of Health; 2023. https://www.ncbi.nlm.nih.gov.
6. CDC. Tetanus. Centers for Disease Control and Prevention; 2023. https://www.cdc.gov.
7. WHO. Tetanus. World Health Organization; 2023. https://www.who.int.
8. National Vaccine Information Center. What is the history of tetanus in America and other countries? Vienna: National Vaccine Information Center; 2022. https://www.nvic.org.
9. NIH. Tetanus. National Institutes of Health Office of NIH History & Stetten Museum; Undated. https://history.nih.gov.
10. Kaufmann SHE. Remembering Emile von Behring: from tetanus treatment to antibody cooperation with phagocytes. MBio. 2017;8(1):e00117. https://www.ncbi.nlm.nih.gov.
11. NIH. Tetanus immune globulin (human): HyperTET®. New York: National Institutes of Health; 2023. https://dailymed.nlm.nih.gov.

Anthrax

12. DOL. Anthrax. U.S. Department of Labor: Occupational Safety and Health Administration; Undated. https://osha.gov/anthrax.
13. CDC. Anthrax: what is anthrax? Centers for Disease Control and Prevention; 2020. https://www.cdc.gov.
14. Friebe S, Gisou van der Goot F, Bürgi J. The ins and outs of anthrax toxin. Toxins. 2016;8(3):69. https://www.ncbi.nlm.nih.gov.
15. Mayo Clinic. Anthrax: symptoms and causes. Jacksonville: Mayo Clinic; 2023. https://www.mayoclinic.org.
16. Editors Encyclopedia Britannica. Anthrax: encyclopedia Britannica. 2023. https://www.britannica.com.
17. Gruno R, Verbeek L, Jacob D, et al. Injection anthrax—a new outbreak in heroin users. Dtsch Arztebl Int. 2012;109(49):843–8. https://www.ncbi.nlm.nih.gov.
18. Turnbull P. Obituary: Max Sterne. The Independent. 1997. https://www.independent.co.uk.
19. Mayo Clinic. Anthrax: diagnosis and treatment. Jacksonville: Mayo Clinic; 2022. https://www.mayoclinic.org.
20. Hesse EM, Godfred-Cato S, Bower WA. Antitoxin use in the prevention and treatment of anthrax disease: a systematic review. Clin Infect Dis. 2002;75(3):432–40. https://academic.oup.com.
21. FDA. Vaccines: anthrax. Silver Spring: U.S. Food and Drug Administration; 2023. https://www.fda.gov.
22. CDC. Anthrax: vaccine to prevent anthrax. Centers for Disease Control and Prevention; 2020. https://www.cdc.gov.

23. ASPR. Stockpile responses. Silver Spring: U.S Department of Health and Human Services: Administration for Strategic Preparedness & Response; Updated 2022. https://aspr.hhs.gov.
24. FBI. Amerithrax or anthrax investigation. Federal Bureau of Investigation; Undated. https://www.fbi.gov.
25. U.S. Department of State. Biological weapons convention. Undated. https://www.state.gov.

Clostridial Myonecrosis

26. Huynh UVP, Nguyen PM, Brusch JL, chief editor. Gas gangrene (clostridial myonecrosis). Medscape. 2023. https://emedicine.medscape.com.
27. Yildiz T, Gündeş S, Willke A, et al. Spontaneous, nontraumatic gas gangrene due to *Clostridium perfringens*. Int J Infect Dis. 2006;10(1):83–5. https://www.ijidonline.com.
28. Buboltz JB, Murphy-Lavoie HM. Gas gangrene. In: StatPearls. New York: National Institutes of Health; 2023. https://www.ncbi.nlm.nih.gov.
29. Bush LM. Gas gangrene (clostridial myonecrosis). Merck Manual: consumer version. 2023. https://www.merckmanuals.com.
30. Cleveland Clinic. Gas gangrene: causes, symptoms, treatment & prevention. Cleveland Clinic; 2023. https://myclevelandclinic.org.

Index